There Are No Cave Drawings of Chairs

A Primal Guide To Posture, Power, And Pain-Free Living

Dr. Chada

There Are No Cave Drawings of Chairs

Copyright © 2025 Primitive Truth

All rights reserved.

No portion of this book may be reproduced in any form without written permission from the publisher or author, except as permitted by U.S. copyright law.

This publication is designed to provide accurate and authoritative information in regard to the subject matter covered. It is sold with the understanding that neither the author nor the publisher is engaged in rendering legal, investment, accounting or other professional services. While the publisher and author have used their best efforts in preparing this book, they make no representations or warranties with respect to the accuracy or completeness of the contents of this book and specifically disclaim any implied warranties of merchantability or fitness for a particular purpose. No warranty may be created or extended by sales representatives or written sales materials. The advice and strategies contained herein may not be suitable for your situation. You should consult with a professional when appropriate. Neither the publisher nor the author shall be liable for any loss of profit or any other commercial damages, including but not limited to special, incidental, consequential, personal, or other damages.

10 9 8 7 6 5 4 3 2 1

First edition 2025

ISBN: 979-8-9991653-0-5 (Paperback)

ISBN: 979-8-9991653-1-2 (Hardcover)

Imprint: Primitive Truth

Printed in the United States of America

DEDICATION

To my chosen, and to my patients, for my reason to live and be better.

SIGN UP FOR AUTHOR UPDATES

Visit http://www.ThereAreNoCaveDrawings.com to:

Sign up for updates: Be the first to know about new articles, insights, and resources related to natural movement, posture, squatting, and holistic health.

Learn about events: Find out about upcoming workshops, webinars, talks, or local events (in Colorado, and beyond!) where I may be speaking or attending.

Access additional resources: Discover curated information, potential blog posts expanding on the topics covered in this book, and news about future projects.

Connect: Find ways to engage further with this important conversation.

Table of Contents

Preface v
Why Are There No Cave Drawings of Chairs?.. 1
Our Ancestors Did Not Need Furniture 7
From Sittin' to Shittin' 16
A Note to the Reader 25
Built to Bend 28
The Elastic Body 36
The Dis-ease Of Sitting 45
Reclaiming Your Natural Nature 53
Primal Birth as Nature Intended 61
A Practical Guide to Reclaiming the Squat 69
Beyond the Chair 80
Bonus Chapter: The Gravity-Assisted Stretch 87
Bonus Chapter II: When You Shoes you Lose 94
About the Author ii
Appendix I - Glossary of Terms iii
Appendix II - Understanding Positions and Directions xi
Pop Quiz iii
Stay Connected! xii

Preface

"I am not looking to go against any belief system. We were either created to be cavemen or we evolved to be cavemen – either way, let us start there."

If you have picked up this book, you, or someone you care about, has experienced the nagging discomfort of low back pain, stiffness in your hips, or general physical limitations that seem to creep in as we navigate modern life. Believe me, I understand. My own journey into the importance of the squat, and the often-overlooked impact of how we sit, began not just in textbooks, but within my own body.

For decades, my professional life involved standing for long hours as a butcher. While physically demanding in its own way, it did not prepare me for the musculoskeletal challenges that arose later. It was not until I embarked on my chiropractic education, trading hours on my feet for hours in chairs listening to lectures, that my own low back and hips began to protest loudly. The simple act of sitting, day after day, began to wreak havoc in a way that years of standing never had. My own body became my first, and perhaps most persistent, puzzle.

An early lesson came when I realized that roughly 20% of my discomfort stemmed from sitting on my wallet! Removing it brought noticeable relief, highlighting how even small, habitual asymmetries could have significant effects. That simple fix, however, was just the beginning.

As I transitioned into private practice here in Colorado, a clear pattern appeared among the people I served. Regardless of age, occupation, or background, nearly everyone showed some level of movement restriction, particularly in the hips, knees, and ankles – the very areas essential for squatting. I saw the consequences daily: pain, stiffness, reduced function, and often, a sense of frustration.

My chiropractic training had equipped me with the tools for analyzing structure and restoring joint function through manipulation. It provided me with the knowledge to seek the structural root cause of any sign or symptom. Yet, I found myself increasingly aware that adjusting joints, while crucial, was not always the complete solution. People felt better, but the underlying patterns related to how they lived, worked, and especially sat, often persisted, or returned. I felt an obligation to the people I served – if the existing approaches were not solving the whole problem, I needed to figure out why.

This quest sent me back to the foundations: human anatomy and biomechanics. But this time, I started asking different questions. Not just "How is this structure?" but "How was this structure intended to function?" I began integrating my anatomical knowledge with insights from anthropology and evolutionary biology, exploring how human bodies moved and rested before modern inventions made life supposedly "easier." Before chairs, before sitting on toilets, before cars and desk jobs reshaped our active daily lifestyle.

And that is when the deep squat truly opened my eyes. It was not just an exercise; it was a fundamental human posture. A posture for rest, for work, for elimination, even for birth. Its absence from modern American living, and the simultaneous dominance of the chair, appeared to be a major missing link in understanding and addressing the widespread musculoskeletal issues I saw every day.

This book is the result of that journey. It is a combination of my subjective experiences, clinical observations, and the interplay between our anatomy, our history, and our modern habits. My goal is to share these insights in an accessible way, to help you understand why your body might be feeling the way it does, and to empower you with practical knowledge and tools to reclaim natural movement, alleviate discomfort, and restore vitality.

My sincere hope is that this book illuminates a path toward understanding, and a more vibrant, embodied life for you. Thank you for joining me on this exploration.

Dr. Chada

There Are No Cave Drawings of Chairs

Why Are There No Cave Drawings of Chairs?

"If we were supposed to walk upright, we would be born upright."

Picture this: You are deep within an ancient cave, the air cool and still. By the flickering light of a torch, you see images painted onto the stone walls thousands of years ago. There are powerful bison, graceful deer, scenes of the hunt, outlines of human hands reaching out from the past. These drawings tell stories of survival, of reverence for nature, of the daily lives of our distant ancestors.

Now, look closer. Scan every image, every symbol. What do you not see?

You do not see anyone lounging in a recliner. You do not see a family gathered around a dining table on matching seats. You do not see a single depiction of what many of us spend a third or even half of our waking lives doing: sitting in a chair.

Dr. Chada

Does that not seem odd to you?

This simple observation is the seed from which this book grows. If chairs are such a normal, necessary part of human life today, why is there absolutely no evidence of them – not even a primitive stool – in the vast records left by early humans? Why are there no cave drawings of chairs?

The answer, which we will explore together throughout these pages, is profoundly simple yet revolutionary in our modern context: Chair-sitting, as we know it, is not a fundamentally natural human posture. It is a relatively recent invention, a piece of cultural furniture we have adopted so completely that we have forgotten the way our bodies were designed to rest and move.

The Original Squat

Think about your very first posture. Long before you took your first breath, curled up safely within the womb, how were you positioned? You were in the fetal position – knees tucked tightly towards your chest, spine gently rounded, head nestled downwards. Look closely at that shape. It is essentially a deep, passive squat.

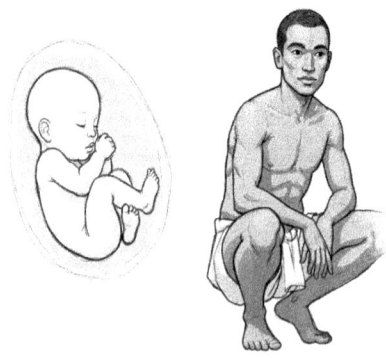

There Are No Cave Drawings of Chairs

This is not a coincidence. It is our biological starting point. We spend months developing in this primal posture. If human beings were fundamentally designed to be rigidly upright from day one, our development should reflect that, right? The fact that we begin life in a flexed, squat-like position hints at something deep within our anatomical blueprint. We are born from this position, and arguably, born for it in many ways.

Intuitive Movement

Watch any healthy toddler who has yet to be influenced by adult furniture and habits. When they want to examine something on the ground, pick up a toy, or simply rest for a moment, what do they do? Effortlessly, with perfect form, they drop into a deep squat. Their heels stay grounded, their backs stay relatively straight, their hips sink below their knees. They can play like this, rest like this, see the world like this for extended periods, comfortably and stable.

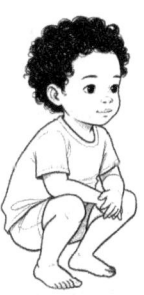

There is no instruction manual needed. They do not need coaching on form. It is an innate, intuitive movement pattern. It is only later, as they begin to mimic the adults around them and are introduced to chairs at home, in daycare, and at school, that this natural ability often starts to fade. They learn to sit up in chairs, often contorting their bodies into positions that compromise the natural curves of their spine and tighten their hips – something we will delve into deeply in Chapters 4 and 5 when we discuss anatomy.

Squatting is Function

The significance of the squat extends far beyond just resting. Think about fundamental human activities throughout history and across cultures:

Giving Birth: As we will explore in detail in Chapter 8, squatting or positions like hands-and-knees are physiologically advantageous for childbirth, opening the pelvic outlet and using gravity. Many traditional cultures intuitively understood this.

Elimination: For much of human history, and still today for billions of people, squatting is the natural posture for bowel movements. The design of the squat toilet aligns with our internal anatomy to allow for more complete and less strained elimination, a topic relevant to the digestive benefits we discuss in Chapter 7.

Work: Consider tasks like tending a fire, gathering food, preparing meals on the ground, planting crops, or crafting tools. Many essential human activities were historically performed from a squat or kneeling position.

Social Interaction: In countless cultures, gathering socially meant sitting or squatting together on the ground, fostering a different kind of connection than sitting rigidly opposite each other in chairs.

Intimacy: Even many natural positions for sexual intimacy involve squat-like mechanics, flexing the hips and knees in ways that are fundamental to our movement capabilities.

Squatting, therefore, is not just one way to be; it is woven into the very fabric of human function, health, and experience. It is a posture of rest, work, birth, and connection.

There Are No Cave Drawings of Chairs

Comfortably Uncomfortable

So, if squatting is so natural, so fundamental, why are we dedicating a whole book to it? Because in our modern, Westernized world, we have lost it. We have traded the dynamic potential of the squat for the static convenience of the chair.

We sit in chairs to eat, to work, to travel, to socialize, to relax. Our homes, schools, offices, and vehicles are designed around the assumption that we will be sitting in chairs. We have become so accustomed to it that the absence of a chair often feels awkward or uncomfortable. For many modern adults, trying a deep squat like the toddler we pictured earlier is difficult, unstable, or even painful. The muscles are too tight, the joints too stiff, the balance unfamiliar.

This book is born from my experience as a Doctor of Chiropractic, not only specializing in, but having a personal passion for human anatomy and musculoskeletal biomechanics. Day after day, I see patients struggling with back pain, hip immobility, neck tension, pelvic floor issues, and a host of other problems often linked to or exacerbated by one major factor: the way we sit, and more importantly, the way we do not move.

Our bodies are crying out for the varied movement, the deep flexion, the natural alignment that postures like squatting provide. Instead, we subject them to hours upon hours of static compression in chairs, often poorly designed ones, leading to predictable patterns of dysfunction. We start to believe that aches, pains, and stiffness are just inevitable parts of aging or modern life. I am here to tell you that, in many cases, they are not inevitable – they are the result of abandoning our natural movement heritage.

What This Book Will Offer You

My goal is not to demand that you throw away all your chairs and live a life exclusively on the floor (though you might find yourself wanting to spend more time there!). Rather, this book aims to:

Open Your Eyes: Help you see chair-sitting not as a default, but as one specific option with significant consequences, contrasting it with our evolutionary norm (Chapters 2 & 3).

Explain the "Why": Dive into the fascinating anatomy and biomechanics of squatting versus chair-sitting, explaining how these postures affect your joints, muscles, spine, and even pelvic floor health in an accessible way (Chapters 4 & 5).

Highlight the Cost: Clearly outline the documented downsides of excessive chair-sitting – the "sitting disease" – and how it contributes to common health complaints (Chapter 6).

Reveal the Benefits: Explore the wide-ranging positive effects of reclaiming the squat, from improved mobility and digestion to potentially easier childbirth (Chapters 7 & 8).

Provide a Path: Offer practical, safe, and progressive strategies to reintroduce squatting and related movements back into your life, regardless of your current ability (Chapter 9).

We will approach this journey together, translating anatomical concepts into understandable language and actionable advice. We will challenge long-held assumptions and empower you to reconnect with your body's innate wisdom.

The absence of chairs in cave drawings is not just a historical curiosity; it is a clue. It points towards a way of being, moving, and resting that is embedded in our biology. It invites us to question our modern habits and consider whether the chair, designed for comfort, might be contributing to our collective discomfort.

Are you ready to explore this missing posture and unlock its potential for your health and wellness? Let us begin by stepping back in time, long before the first chair was ever conceived.

There Are No Cave Drawings of Chairs

Our Ancestors Did Not Need Furniture

"There are no cave drawings of pillows or mattresses either... Our ancestors lived differently, closer to the earth."

In the last chapter, we stood before imaginary cave walls, noticing the conspicuous absence of chairs in the records left by our ancient ancestors. That absence is not just a quirky detail; it is a doorway into understanding how humans lived, moved, and rested for much of our time on Earth. Forget centuries; we need to think in terms of millennia – hundreds of thousands of years where *Homo sapiens* thrived without a single armchair, office chair, or even a simple three-legged stool in sight.

So, how did they manage? Did they just stand all day? Or lie down whenever they were not actively hunting or gathering? The evidence gathered from studying human history, cultures still living traditional lifestyles, and even our own bones, points overwhelmingly to a different reality: For most of human history, squatting was not just a resting posture; it was the primary resting posture

Living Proof

While we cannot directly observe our Paleolithic ancestors, we can gain valuable insights from studying contemporary hunter-gatherer groups whose lifestyles may echo those of pre-agricultural humans. One of the most studied groups in this context is the Hadza people of Tanzania. They live active lives, foraging for food in the savanna. And when they rest, socialize, or perform tasks near the ground, what do they often do? They squat.

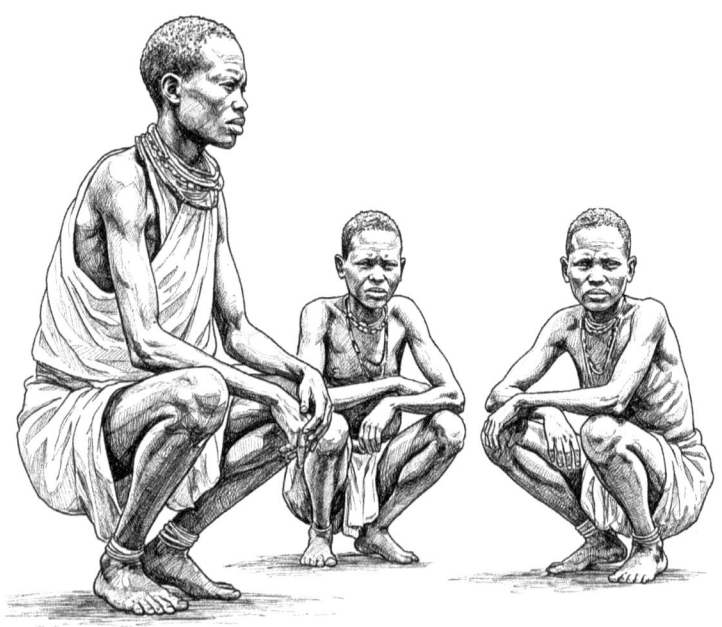

There Are No Cave Drawings of Chairs

Anthropologists observing the Hadza note that both men and women often adopt a deep squat position throughout the day. It is used for resting between bursts of activity, preparing food, tending fires, sharing stories, and keeping watch. It is not seen as strenuous or temporary; it is simply a comfortable, stable, and efficient way to be close to the ground. They transition in and out of it fluidly, showing a level of ease and mobility that might seem extraordinary to many modern, chair-bound individuals.

The Hadza are not unique. Similar patterns of frequent squatting and ground-level living have been observed in many indigenous and traditional cultures around the globe, from parts of Asia to Africa to Central and South America. While specific styles might vary, the underlying principle remains: resting and living close to the earth, utilizing the body's natural ability to fold deeply at the hips, knees, and ankles, was the human norm.

The Skeletal Record

But we do not have to rely solely on observing living cultures. Our own skeletons can hold clues about the habitual movements of our ancestors. When a particular movement or posture is performed often over a lifetime, it can leave subtle marks on the bones as the body adapts.

Physical anthropologists have identified specific features, sometimes called "squatting facets," which are small, smooth areas or modifications on the ankle bones (talus and tibia) and sometimes even the hip joint. These facets are thought to develop in response to the extreme range of motion and pressure experienced during habitual deep squatting, where the shin bone presses firmly against the front of the ankle bone.

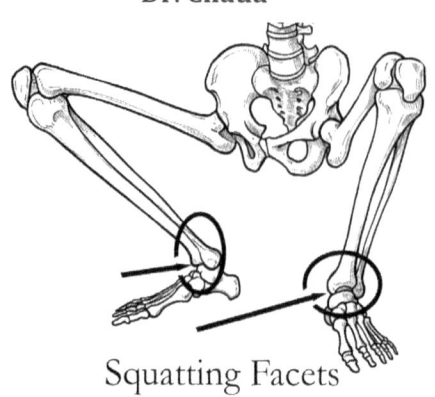

Squatting Facets

The presence of these facets in ancient skeletal remains provides compelling physical evidence that deep squatting was not just an occasional activity but a regular, everyday posture for many past populations. It tells us their bodies adapted to this position because it was so commonplace. Conversely, these facets are often less common or absent in skeletal populations from more recent, industrialized societies where chair-sitting dominates. Our bones tell a story of changing movement habits. As we will explore when we dive into anatomy (Chapters 4 and 5), this habitual deep flexion is precisely what keeps these joints healthy and mobile – a benefit lost when we confine ourselves to the limited range of motion offered by chairs.

The Silence of the Artifacts

Think about the things archaeologists dug up from ancient human settlements. They find stone tools, spear points, pottery shards, beads, remnants of shelters, and evidence of fire pits. These artifacts paint a picture of daily life, of survival, creativity, and community.

Now, consider what is missing from the earliest and longest periods of human history: furniture designed for sitting. While a natural rock or log might certainly have been used opportunistically, purpose-built seats like stools or chairs are

There Are No Cave Drawings of Chairs

remarkably rare until much more recently in the grand scheme of things. If sitting elevated off the ground was a fundamental human need or comfort, would we not expect to find more evidence of early seating innovations among the many other tools and objects our ancestors crafted?

The relative silence of the archaeological record regarding chairs, compared to the abundance of tools for other daily tasks, further supports the idea that ground-level living, incorporating postures like squatting and kneeling, was the standard.

Art Tells a Story (Often on the Ground)

When we look at depictions of daily life from early civilizations – places like ancient Egypt or Mesopotamia – we often see figures working, celebrating, or eating while positioned close to the ground. While pharaohs and gods might be shown on thrones (an early indicator of seating as a status symbol, which we will touch on in Chapter 3), scenes of common people frequently show them kneeling, sitting cross-legged, or performing tasks in a posture that implies squatting, especially for agricultural or craft work.

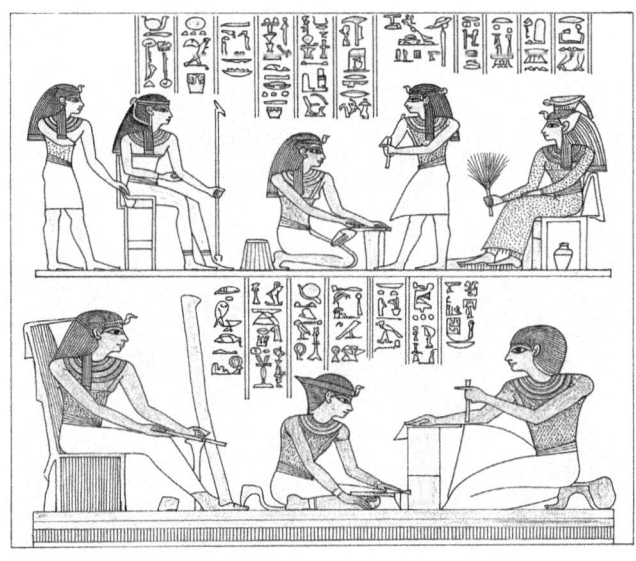

These artistic glimpses reinforce the idea that life was not lived perched on individual chairs but rather engaged at ground level.

The Chair is Young

It is easy to lose sight of just how long humans have existed compared to how long we have had chairs as everyday objects. Let us try an analogy. Imagine the entire history of *Homo sapiens* (roughly 300,000 years) stretched out as a mile-long road.

- For almost the entire length of that mile – thousands upon thousands of feet representing hundreds of thousands of years – people are living without chairs as common items. They are squatting, kneeling, walking, running, resting on the ground.
- Evidence of chairs as status symbols for the elite might appear in the last few hundred feet.
- Chairs becoming somewhat common household items in Western societies? That is perhaps only in the last 50-100 feet of that mile.
- The pervasive, near-constant chair-sitting of modern office work, commuting, and leisure? That reality dominates only the final few inches of our mile-long journey.

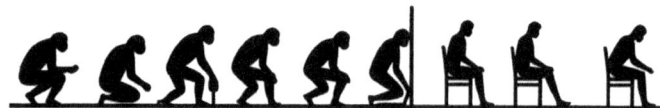

There Are No Cave Drawings of Chairs

This perspective is crucial. It helps us understand that our current relationship with chairs is not the culmination of long-term evolution; it is a very recent, abrupt shift away from millennia of ground-based living. Our bodies, genetically and anatomically, are still largely adapted to that older, more varied movement pattern that included frequent squatting. Is it any wonder they often protest when forced into chairs for hours on end, as we will see in Chapter 6?

The Practical Wisdom of the Squat

Why was squatting such a successful and enduring posture? From a purely practical standpoint, it offered several advantages:

Energy Conservation: Standing requires continuous low-level muscle activation to maintain balance and fight gravity. Lying down is restful but not ideal for staying alert or quickly reacting. Squatting provides a stable resting position that requires less muscular effort than standing, conserving valuable energy, yet keeps a person oriented, alert, and ready to move if needed.

Thermoregulation: Being closer to the ground could be advantageous for warmth, especially around a fire, or potentially for staying cooler in certain hot environments.

Platform for Work: It provides a stable, low base for performing tasks done best at ground level – preparing food, tending crops, crafting tools, playing with children.

It was, quite simply, an efficient, versatile, and biologically appropriate posture for the demands of ancestral life.

A World of Floor Living

It is also important to note that squatting is not the only form of natural human ground-living. Across the globe, cultures developed rich traditions of sitting and kneeling directly on the floor. Think of the Japanese seiza (kneeling with buttocks resting on heels), various cross-legged positions common in South Asia and the Middle East, or side-sitting postures.

These postures, while distinct from a deep squat, share key characteristics: they involve greater flexion at the hips and knees than chair-sitting, they engage different muscles, and they are part of a lifestyle less reliant on elevated furniture. The prevalence of these diverse floor-based customs further underscores the point that chair-sitting is the exception, not the rule, in the broad sweep of human culture and history.

Born Ready

Let us circle back briefly to the image of the toddler we discussed in Chapter 1, effortlessly dropping into that perfect, deep squat.

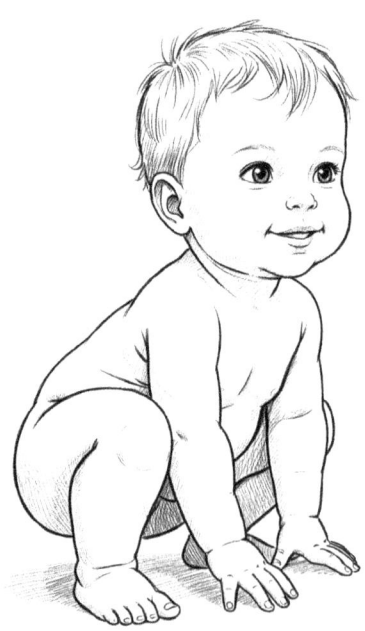

There Are No Cave Drawings of Chairs

This is not a learned behavior; it is an expression of our innate human movement potential. Before cultural conditioning, before spending hours confined to car seats, highchairs, and school desks, our bodies know how to squat. It is woven into our neuromuscular development. The fact that we typically lose this ability as we adopt modern lifestyles speaks volumes about the power of our environment (and our furniture choices) to reshape our physical capabilities, often to our detriment.

History Matters to Your Health

Why spend a whole chapter exploring this history? Because understanding that squatting is our ancestral norm, not some new fitness fad, is fundamental to appreciating its importance for our health and wellness today. It reframes the aches and pains many experience from chronic chair-sitting (which we will dissect in Chapter 6) not as personal failings, but as predictable consequences of abandoning a biologically congruent way of moving and resting.

Our history tells us our bodies were designed to fold, bend, and rest close to the ground. The historical and anthropological evidence strongly suggests that the human frame thrives when it regularly experiences the deep flexion of a squat. By recognizing this, we can begin to see reclaiming the squat not as forcing our bodies into an unnatural position, but as welcoming back a long-lost, vital part of our human movement heritage.

The story does not end here, of course. If squatting was the norm, how did the chair conquer the world? In the next chapter, we will trace the surprising history of the chair itself – from symbol of power to ubiquitous necessity – and explore how its rise contributed to the decline of the squat, setting the stage for many of the musculoskeletal challenges we face today.

Dr. Chada

From Sittin' to Shittin'

"We did not just invent the chair; we invented the need to sit in it, reshaping our world and our bodies in the process."

In the last chapter, we journeyed back through the vast expanse of human history, discovering that for millennia, squatting was not just an option; it was deeply woven into the fabric of daily life as a primary posture for rest, work, and community. Our ancestors, as shown by their bones, their art, and the practices of traditional cultures, lived life closer to the ground. So, if we spent hundreds of thousands of years thriving without dedicated seating furniture, how did we arrive at today's world – a world built, quite literally, around the chair? How did this object, absent from those cave walls we pondered in Chapter 1, rise to such prominence that not using one often feels strange?

There Are No Cave Drawings of Chairs

The story is not one of sudden invention but rather a slow, gradual creep, driven by shifts in social structures, technology, and eventually, our very definition of comfort and necessity. It is a journey from rare symbols of power to ubiquitous items of furniture, culminating in an environment that constantly invites, and often demands, that we sit.

Seats of Power

The earliest known chairs were not designed for the comfort of the masses. They were symbols of status, reserved for the highest echelons of society – rulers, priests, and gods. Think of the elaborate thrones of Egyptian pharaohs or the ceremonial seats depicted in ancient Greek and Roman art.

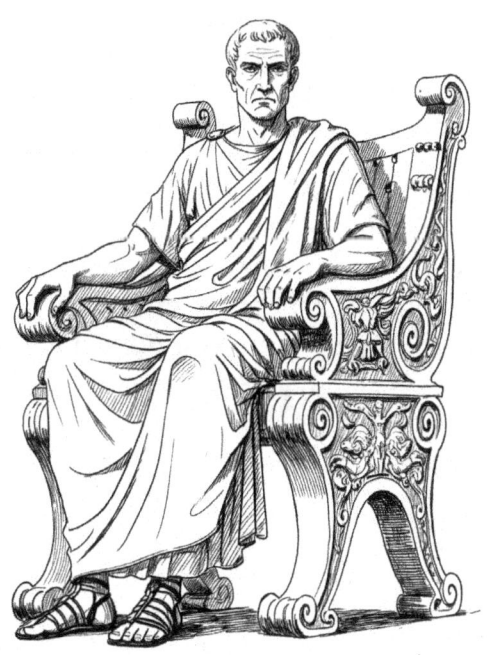

To be seated while others stood or sat on the ground was a clear visual marker of authority and importance. Being physically elevated separated the ruler from the ruled, the divine from the mortal. These early chairs were often ornate, crafted from precious materials, and uncomfortable by modern standards – their purpose was not ergonomic support, but symbolic elevation. For much of the population during these times, life continued at ground level, using the squat, kneeling, or sitting on simple mats or the earth itself, as discussed in Chapter 2. The chair, in its infancy, was an exception, not the rule.

A Slow Trickle Down: Chairs Enter the Home (Slowly)

For centuries following antiquity, the chair remained an uncommon object. Throughout the Middle Ages and even into the Renaissance, while royalty and high clergy kept their imposing seats, common households typically relied on simpler forms of seating, if any dedicated furniture at all. Benches, chests (which doubled as storage and seating), and three-legged stools were more prevalent than individual chairs with backs and arms.

Inside the average home, many activities – cooking, eating, mending, socializing – still occurred closer to the floor or around a central hearth. While chairs gradually became more common in the homes of the growing merchant class and landed gentry from the Renaissance onwards, they were still often considered significant pieces of furniture, not the disposable, ubiquitous items they are today. True democratization of the chair was yet to come.

The Shift

The real turning point in our relationship with sitting arrived with the Industrial Revolution, beginning in the late 18th century. The shift from agrarian and craft-based economies to factory

There Are No Cave Drawings of Chairs

production brought enormous changes to how people worked and lived.

Factory work often required individuals to perform repetitive tasks in one place for hours on end. While early factory conditions were often unpleasant and seating might have been minimal, the nature of the work itself began to normalize prolonged periods of static posture. Simultaneously, the growth of industry fueled the expansion of commerce, administration, and bureaucracy, leading to the birth of the modern office.

Clerks, managers, and administrators spent their days sitting at desks, shuffling papers, writing ledgers, and managing the burgeoning complexities of industrial society. The chair became an essential tool of this new white-collar workforce. This era marked a fundamental shift: prolonged sitting was no longer just the privilege (or burden) of the elite or the occasional choice of the masses; it was becoming an economic necessity for large segments of the population.

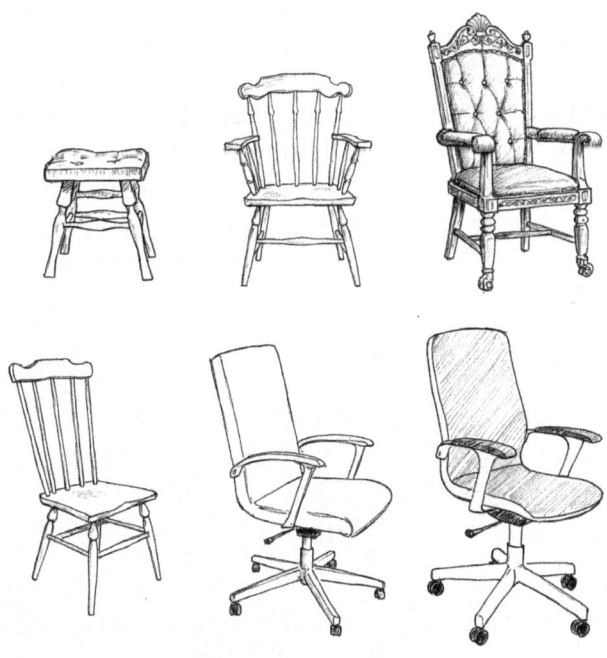

Dr. Chada
Designing Ourselves into Sedentary Habits

As chair use grew, so did the variety and design of chairs themselves. We moved from basic wooden constructions to more elaborate upholstered armchairs, driven by a growing middle class seeking comfort and domestic refinement. The 20th century saw the rise of functionalism and mass production, leading to chairs designed for specific purposes – the typist's chair, the school desk chair, the automobile seat, the airplane seat.

The latter half of the 20th century brought the concept of "ergonomics" – designing objects to optimize human well-being and performance. The ergonomic office chair, with its adjustable lumbar supports, armrests, heights, and tilting mechanisms, promised to solve the problems caused by prolonged sitting. However, as many of us experiencing daily aches and pains can attest, and as we will explore from an anatomical perspective in Chapter 6, even the most expensive ergonomic chair fails to negate the fundamental issue: our bodies are not designed to remain static in any position for hours on end. The very idea of a chair providing perfect, passive support undermines the body's need for movement and the natural engagement of postural muscles that occurs with more dynamic postures like squatting (as detailed in Chapter 5). Often, these ergonomic features simply accommodate or even encourage poor postural habits rather than solving the root problem.

The Most Personal of Seats

Perhaps no single invention cemented the decline of the squat in daily life more profoundly than the widespread adoption of the modern sitting toilet. For millennia, across virtually all cultures, humans squatted to eliminate waste. This posture, as we now understand and will be discussed further in Chapters 5 and 7, naturally aligns the colon and relaxes the puborectalis muscle, allowing for easier and more complete evacuation.

There Are No Cave Drawings of Chairs

The invention of the flush toilet (with early versions appearing much earlier but becoming widespread in the 19th and 20th centuries) prioritized sanitation and convenience over physiological alignment. The seated position on a typical Western toilet places the body at roughly a 90-degree angle at the hips and knees. This keeps the puborectalis muscle partially constricted, effectively kinking the colon and requiring straining to eliminate waste.

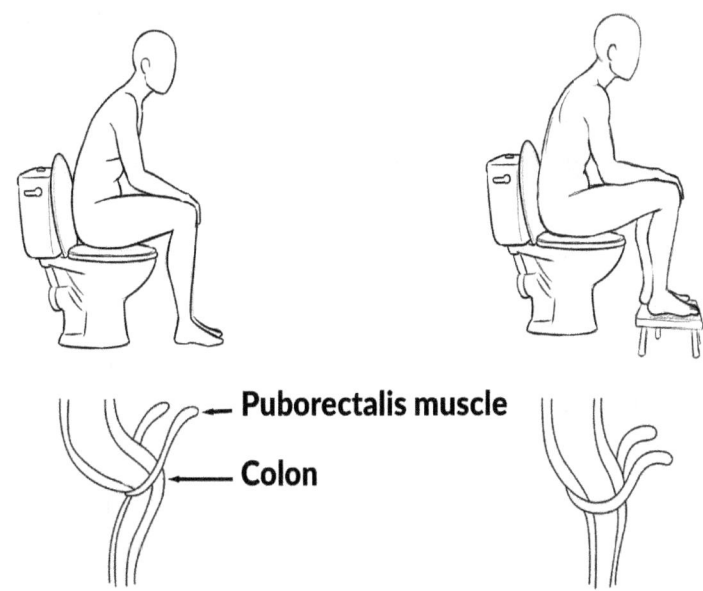

While the flush toilet was a major public health advancement in terms of sanitation, its design inadvertently pushed aside a fundamental, physiologically optimal human posture. Billions of people worldwide still use squat toilets today, and the rise of constipation, hemorrhoids, and other colorectal issues in Western societies has led some to question the wisdom of abandoning the squat for this daily biological function. Devices like the Squatty Potty® or simple footstools aim to help users mimic a more squat-like angle even on a sitting toilet, implicitly acknowledging the biomechanical sense of the older posture. The toilet, arguably the most personal chair we use, fundamentally altered a primal human movement pattern.

Building Our World Around the Chair

Once chairs became common, our environment started to reshape itself around them. Think about it:

Table and Desk Heights: Standard heights assume a person will be sitting in a chair of a certain height. Working or eating at these surfaces while squatting or kneeling is often awkward or impossible.

Classroom Design: Rows of desks and chairs became the norm, training children from a young age to sit still for extended periods.

Transportation: Cars, trains, buses, and airplanes are designed entirely around seated passengers.

Homes: Living rooms center around sofas and armchairs facing a television; dining rooms feature tables and chairs. Even kitchen counter heights often presume a standing or stool-seated user.

Public Spaces: Waiting rooms, theaters, stadiums, restaurants – all are filled with chairs, reinforcing sitting as the default public posture.

This pervasive environmental design creates a feedback loop. Because the environment is built for chairs, we use chairs. And because we use chairs, we continue to build environments that necessitate them. Opting out of chair-use requires conscious effort and often modification of one's surroundings; it goes against the grain of modern design.

The Allure of Convenience

Why did we embrace the chair so readily? Part of the appeal is undoubtedly perceived comfort and convenience. Especially for individuals who have lost the mobility required for easy squatting

There Are No Cave Drawings of Chairs

(often due to a lifetime of chair use!), sitting down feels easier. It requires less flexibility, less balance, and less muscular effort in the moment.

But this convenience comes at a cost. By constantly outsourcing the work of supporting our body weight to an external object (the chair), we engage in a form of physical de-skilling. The muscles designed to hold us upright, stabilize our core, and maintain posture – muscles that are active and coordinated in a squat (as we will see in Chapter 5) – become passive, weak, and imbalanced from chronic chair-sitting. The connective tissues and joints lose their healthy range of motion through disuse.

We have traded the active, dynamic stability of natural postures like the squat for the passive, static support of furniture. This trade might seem comfortable initially, but it leaves our bodies unprepared for movement, prone to injury, and susceptible to the host of problems associated with the "sitting disease" (Chapter 6).

A Historical Hangover

Our journey through the history of the chair reveals that our current sitting habits are not an evolutionary inevitability but a relatively recent historical development. We moved from a world where squatting was the norm and chairs were rare symbols of power, to a world where chairs are ubiquitous, and squatting feels alien to many. This transition, driven by social change, industrialization, and technological innovation like the sitting toilet, has profoundly reshaped our bodies and our health.

Understanding this history is crucial. It helps us recognize that the way we live now is not the only way, nor necessarily the best way, for our bodies, which still carry the anatomical legacy of those ancestors who did not need furniture. This historical "hangover" – the mismatch between our ancient biology and our modern sitting habits – is a key factor in many contemporary health challenges.

Dr. Chada

Now that we have seen how the chair rose to prominence, we need to understand what this shift means for our physical structures. In the next chapters, we will dive deep into the fascinating mechanics of your own body, exploring the anatomy of the squat versus the chair-sit, and uncovering exactly why reclaiming that ancestral posture can be so beneficial for your health and vitality today.

There Are No Cave Drawings of Chairs

A Note to the Reader

Bringing Anatomy and Movement to Life

As we transition from exploring the history of sitting and squatting into the fascinating details of our own bodies, we encounter concepts that are often best understood visually and dynamically. While illustrations in a book are helpful, seeing anatomy in motion and watching demonstrations of specific movements can significantly deepen your understanding and confidence.

To provide you with this richer learning experience, starting in the next chapter, you will find special QR codes embedded within the text, like the example below:

Scan To Meet Me!

What is a QR Code?

Think of a QR code (Quick Response code) as a type of barcode that your smartphone or tablet camera can read. When scanned, it acts like a direct link, instantly taking you to a specific webpage, video, or other online resource.

How to Use the QR Codes in This Book:

- **Open Your Camera App**: On most modern smartphones or tablets, simply open the built-in camera application.
- **Point at the Code**: Aim your camera at the QR code printed in the book, as if you were going to take a picture of it. Hold steady for a moment.
- **Tap the Link**: Your device should automatically recognize the code and display a notification or link on your screen. Tap this link.
- **Watch the Video**: You will be taken directly to a short video hosted online. These videos, created specifically for this book, will feature visual explanations of the anatomical concepts being discussed or clear demonstrations of the movements and exercises described.

(Note: If your camera app does not automatically scan QR codes, you may need to download a free QR code reader app from your device's app store.)

Why Videos? More Than Just Visuals

My goal with this book is to empower you not just with knowledge but with practical ability. Seeing the joints move, understanding how muscles engage, and watching correct form for exercises like the squat progressions (Chapter 9) or the gravity-assisted stretch (Bonus Chapter I) can make all the difference in applying these concepts safely and effectively in your own body.

There Are No Cave Drawings of Chairs

These video supplements are designed to enhance, not replace, the text. They offer a dynamic visual layer to help solidify your understanding and guide your practice.

Connecting Beyond the Page

Furthermore, these videos offer a chance for us to connect more directly. You will not only see the concepts demonstrated, but you will also see and hear me, Dr. Chada, explaining them personally, just as I might in my clinic. Think of it as bringing a bit of that interactive learning experience right to you.

Depending on the platform hosting the videos (currently ThereAreNoCaveDrawings.com), you may also find opportunities to engage further – perhaps by leaving comments or asking clarifying questions related to the video content. This adds another layer to your learning, allowing for interaction that goes beyond the static page.

I encourage you to utilize these QR codes as you encounter them in the upcoming chapters. Let's bring this information off the page and into living motion, fostering both deeper understanding and a stronger connection!

Now, let's dive into the incredible design of your skeleton...

Dr. Chada

Built to Bend

"Nobody has ever blown a knee muscle. There are no muscles in the front or the back of the knee to stop it from bending, only you (or injury).

In the last chapter, we traced the surprising journey of the chair, from a rare symbol of power to an object that dictates much of our modern posture. We saw how historical shifts and technological changes, like the sitting toilet, nudged us away from the ground-level living that characterized most of human history (Chapter 2). But history only tells part of the story. To truly understand why this shift matters to our health and well-being, we need to look inward – at the incredible structure that supports us: our skeleton.

Many people think of the skeleton as just a rigid frame, like the studs inside a wall. But it is so much more than that. It is a living, dynamic system, constantly adapting, and brilliantly designed for a wide range of movements. And as we will explore now, the deep squat is not some extreme or unnatural contortion; it is a posture that beautifully utilizes the inherent capabilities built into our bones and joints. Forget the idea that we are meant to be stiff and upright all the time; we are, quite literally, built to bend.

The Hip Joints: Ball-and-Socket Brilliance

Let's start with the hips, the crucial link between your torso and your legs. Each hip joint is a classic "ball-and-socket" joint. Imagine the rounded head of your thigh bone (femur) – the "ball" – fitting snugly into a cup-like depression in your pelvis (the acetabulum) – the "socket."

This ball-and-socket design is ingenious because it allows for movement in multiple directions: forward (flexion, like bringing your knee towards your chest), backward (extension), sideways (abduction/adduction), and rotation (turning your leg in or out). A deep squat primarily involves significant hip flexion.

Now, you might worry, "Does not folding that deeply pinch something in the front of the hip?" While pinching (known as impingement) can happen, it is often related to stiffness, muscle imbalances, or specific anatomical variations. A healthy hip joint, moved correctly, has ample space to allow the thigh bone to glide smoothly into deep flexion without bone hitting bone painfully. In fact, moving the hip through this full range, as achieved in a proper squat, is essential for maintaining the health and mobility of the joint capsule and surrounding tissues.

Contrast this with sitting in a chair. Your hips are typically fixed at roughly 90 degrees of flexion for prolonged periods. This static position offers none of the range-of-motion benefits of a squat. Over time, the tissues at the front of the hip can become chronically shortened and tight, while the joint itself rarely experiences its full potential movement, contributing to stiffness and sometimes even that pinching sensation when you later try to flex deeply. The squat invites the hip joint to express its full, brilliant design; the chair often restricts it.

The Knees: Nourishing the Hinge

Moving down the leg, we arrive at the knees. Primarily, the knee acts like a hinge, allowing your lower leg to swing backward (flexion) and forward (extension). It also has a small amount of rotational ability, crucial for smooth movement. Inside the knee joint, the ends of the thigh bone (femur) and shin bone (tibia) are covered with smooth, slippery articular cartilage. Between them sit two C-shaped pads of tougher cartilage called menisci, acting as shock absorbers and stabilizers.

Cartilage is fascinating stuff. Unlike most tissues in your body, it does not have a direct blood supply. So, how does it get nutrients and get rid of waste products? Through movement! Specifically,

There Are No Cave Drawings of Chairs

through cycles of compression and release. Think of the cartilage like a kitchen sponge. When you squat deeply, you fully flex the knee, gently compressing the cartilage and squeezing out old synovial fluid (the joint's natural lubricant) and waste products. As you stand back up, the pressure releases, and the cartilage "soaks up" fresh, nutrient-rich synovial fluid.

A deep squat takes the knee through its maximum natural range of flexion, ensuring that all parts of the cartilage get this beneficial "squeeze and soak" cycle. Chair sitting, again, typically locks the knee at around 90 degrees. This means only a limited portion of the cartilage experiences significant pressure changes, potentially leading to malnourishment and degeneration in other areas over time. Furthermore, the lack of full flexion can contribute to stiffness in the joint capsule and surrounding muscles (which we will cover in Chapter 5). The squat does not just bend the knee; it actively nourishes it.

The Ankles: The Flexible Foundation

Often overlooked, the ankle joint is critical for a healthy squat and overall movement. The ability to bend the ankle so that the top of your foot moves towards your shin is called dorsiflexion. Achieving a deep squat with your heels flat on the ground requires a significant amount of ankle dorsiflexion.

Why is this so important? If your ankles are stiff and lack dorsiflexion (a very common issue in modern populations, partly due to lack of use and footwear like high heels), your body must compensate when you try to squat. You might find your heels lifting off the ground, forcing more weight onto the balls of your feet and knees. Or you might compensate by excessively rounding your lower back or leaning your torso too far forward, putting strain elsewhere.

Healthy ankle mobility allows your shins to travel forward over your feet during a squat, keeping your center of gravity balanced and enabling your hips and knees to reach their full depth without undue strain. Like the hips and knees, the ankle joints benefit from being moved through their full range, maintaining the health of the joint capsule and surrounding tissues. Regular squatting is one of the best ways to preserve or gently restore this vital ankle flexibility, which also plays a role in the health of your foot arches and your overall balance.

Maintaining the Natural Curves

Now, let's consider the pillar of our skeleton: the spine. Your spine is not a rigid rod; it is a marvel of engineering with natural curves that help absorb shock and distribute forces. Viewed from the side, you have an inward curve in your neck (cervical lordosis), an outward curve in your mid-back (thoracic kyphosis), and another inward curve in your lower back (lumbar lordosis).

When you perform a squat with good form, the goal is to maintain these natural spinal curves as much as possible, especially

There Are No Cave Drawings of Chairs

the lumbar lordosis. This allows the strong muscles of your back and core (discussed in Chapter 5) to stabilize your torso effectively, and it distributes the load more evenly across the spinal vertebrae and discs.

Contrast this with the posture many people adopt almost unconsciously when sitting in a chair, especially when fatigued or leaning forward towards a desk or screen. The pelvis often tilts backward, causing the lower back to round outwards, reversing the natural lumbar curve into a "C-slump." This posture puts significant pressure on the spinal discs, particularly in the lower back, stretches the ligaments, and deactivates the core muscles that should be providing support. Over time, this can contribute significantly to low back pain, disc issues, and postural dysfunction – common complaints we will address in Chapter 6. While a squat requires active effort to maintain spinal alignment, it respects the spine's natural design; passive chair-slouching often directly opposes it.

Motion is Lotion

There is a common phrase in movement circles: "Motion is lotion." This perfectly captures the principle of joint health we touched upon with the knees. Synovial fluid, that vital lubricant within our joints, circulates nutrients and removes waste products most effectively when the joint is moved through its full available range of motion.

Think about it: if you only ever bend your elbow halfway, the parts of the joint surface that only make contact during full bending or full straightening do not get the same flushing and nourishment. Over time, this can lead to stiffness and degeneration. The same applies to your hips, knees, and ankles.

Squatting is a compound movement – it involves multiple joints moving through a broad range simultaneously. This makes it incredibly efficient at promoting this "motion is lotion" effect throughout the lower body. It ensures that the joint surfaces glide across each other, stimulating synovial fluid production and circulation, and helping to keep the cartilage healthy and resilient. Chair sitting, involving minimal movement and static mid-range positions, starves our joints of this vital nourishment.

Use It or Lose It

Our bodies are masters of adaptation. If we consistently ask them to perform a certain movement, they get better at it. Conversely, if we consistently avoid moving into certain ranges, the body adapts by tightening up and restricting that movement. This "use it or lose it" principle absolutely applies to joint range of motion.

The comfortable, deep squat requires significant flexibility in the hips, knees, and ankles. If you spend years primarily moving within the limited ranges required by walking and chair-sitting, the muscles, ligaments, and joint capsules surrounding these joints will gradually shorten and stiffen, physically limiting your ability to squat deeply.

Reintroducing squatting (gradually and safely, as we will guide you in Chapter 9) is a powerful way to reclaim this lost range of motion. It gently encourages tissues to lengthen and joints to move towards their end ranges, restoring the mobility that our skeleton was inherently designed to possess. It is not about forcing anything; it is about reminding your body of its innate capabilities.

The Skeletal Symphony

It is crucial to see the squat not just as individual joint actions but as a coordinated symphony. The mobility of your ankles affects how well your knees can track and how deep your hips can go. The position of your hips influences the curve of your spine. Stiffness or restriction in one area will inevitably cause compensation in another.

When all parts are working well – flexible ankles, mobile hips, stable knees, and a well-aligned spine – the squat becomes a smooth, efficient, and safe movement that distributes forces appropriately. Problems arise when one part of this kinetic chain is compromised, often due to the lack of movement diversity fostered by chair-dependent lifestyles.

The Cost of Sitting

So, to briefly summarize the skeletal implications of chronic chair sitting versus squatting:

Chair Sitting: Promotes joint stiffness (limited range, poor fluid exchange), encourages poor spinal posture (C-slump, increased disc load), may contribute to hip joint tightness/impingement.

Squatting: Encourages full joint range of motion, nourishes cartilage via fluid exchange, promotes healthy spinal alignment, maintains hip/knee/ankle mobility.

Understanding this skeletal foundation is key to appreciating why common aches and pains – stiff hips, sore knees, aching backs – might not just be random misfortune or inevitable aging. They can often be the logical consequence of systematically denying our skeleton the kind of movement it was designed for, the kind embodied in the deep squat.

Our bones provide the structure, the framework upon which movement happens. They are brilliantly designed for dynamic life. In the next chapter, we will clothe this skeleton, exploring the muscles, fascia, and crucial pelvic floor – the elastic tissues that power our movement and are profoundly affected by our choice of posture.

Dr. Chada

The Elastic Body

"Bones provide the frame, but our elastic tissues grant us movement. Neglect them, and the frame stiffens."

In Chapter 4, we marveled at the design of our skeleton – a structure truly "built to bend." We saw how the shapes of our hip, knee, and ankle joints, and the natural curves of our spine, are perfectly suited for deep movements like the squat. But bones alone do no create movement. They are the levers and framework, brought to life by an intricate network of elastic tissues: muscles that contract and lengthen, fascia that connects and supports, and the vital muscular sling at the base of our core – the pelvic floor.

Think of your body less like a rigid statue and more like a responsive, adaptable structure – strong where it needs to be, yet flexible and yielding where required. This chapter explores how the

There Are No Cave Drawings of Chairs

simple act of squatting engages and cultivates this healthy elasticity, while prolonged chair-sitting often does the opposite, creating patterns of tension, weakness, and imbalance that can lead to discomfort and dysfunction.

The Movers: Muscles That Power the Squat

When you lower yourself into a squat and stand back up, a whole team of muscles works in beautiful coordination. Let's meet the main players:

Quadriceps (Front Thigh): This group of four muscles runs down the front of your thigh. As you lower into a squat (the eccentric phase), your quads work like brakes, controlling the speed of your descent against gravity. As you stand back up (the concentric phase), they contract powerfully to straighten your knees.

Gluteus Maximus (Your Buttocks): This is the largest muscle in your body, and for good reason! It is a primary mover when it comes to extending your hips – think standing up from a squat or chair, climbing stairs, or running. In a deep squat, the glutes are stretched at the bottom and then fire powerfully to help drive you upwards. Engaging your glutes properly is crucial for protecting your lower back.

Hamstrings (Back Thigh): These muscles run down the back of your thigh and cross both the hip and knee joints. They work alongside the glutes to extend the hips and also help stabilize the knee during the squat movement.

Core Muscles (The Stabilizing Canister): This is critical, and it is much more than just your "six-pack" abs! Think of your core as a strong, supportive cylinder.

The deep abdominal muscles (like the Transversus Abdominis) wrap around you like a corset.

The back extensor muscles (like the Erector Spinae) run along your spine.

The Diaphragm (your primary breathing muscle) forms the roof.

The Pelvic Floor muscles (more on these soon!) form the base. When you squat, especially with any added load, these core muscles should engage synergistically – working together to create internal pressure (intra-abdominal pressure) that stabilizes your spine, protecting it from excessive strain much like an inflated canister resists crushing forces.

Activating these large muscle groups through their full range, as happens in a squat, is essential for building functional strength – the kind of strength you need for everyday activities, from lifting groceries to playing with grandkids.

The Yielders: Muscles That Lengthen in the Squat

Movement is not just about contraction; it is also about letting go. For you to sink into a deep squat, several key muscle groups need to lengthen appropriately:

Hip Flexors (Front of Hip): This group includes muscles like the psoas and iliacus, which lift your knee towards your chest. Because many of us spend hours sitting with these muscles in a shortened position, they often become chronically tight. The deep

There Are No Cave Drawings of Chairs

hip flexion required by a squat provides a natural, active stretch for these muscles, helping to counteract the effects of prolonged sitting.

Adductors (Inner Thigh): These muscles draw your legs together. Depending on your squat stance (how wide your feet are), the adductors often need to lengthen to allow your knees to track outwards slightly, making space for your torso to descend between your thighs.

Calves (Back of Lower Leg): As we discussed in Chapter 4 regarding ankle mobility, the calf muscles (Gastrocnemius and Soleus) must lengthen sufficiently to allow your shin to move forward over your foot (dorsiflexion). Tight calves are a very common barrier to achieving a deep, flat-footed squat.

Low Back Extensors: While these muscles work to stabilize the spine (as mentioned above), achieving the very bottom position of a squat can sometimes involve a slight, controlled relaxation or lengthening, offering a gentle counter-stretch to the compression these muscles might experience during prolonged standing or sitting with poor posture.

The squat, therefore, is a beautiful balance of effort and ease – some muscles work hard while others yield and lengthen, all in coordination.

The Chair's Legacy

Now, let's contrast this dynamic interplay with the typical state induced by chronic chair-sitting. Instead of balanced activation and lengthening, sitting often creates predictable imbalances:

Tight Hip Flexors: Hours spent with hips flexed at 90 degrees leads to adaptive shortening.

Weak/Inactive Glutes: When you sit on your glutes, they are not required to work. They can become weak and "forget" how to activate properly – a condition sometimes called "gluteal amnesia." Weak glutes often mean other muscles (like hamstrings or low back muscles) must compensate for them and become overworked.

Deactivated Core: Slouching in a chair turns off the deep core muscles that should be stabilizing your spine.

Tight Hamstrings: While sitting shortens hip flexors, it can paradoxically lead to a feeling of hamstring tightness, partly due to pelvic positioning and neural tension.

Think of your muscles working in pairs around joints, like sets of rubber bands. If one side becomes chronically tight (like the hip flexors from sitting), the opposing side (the glutes) becomes relatively lengthened and weak. This imbalance pulls on your bones and joints (like your pelvis and spine), altering your posture and movement patterns, and setting the stage for pain and injury. These common imbalances are often major contributors to the low back pain, hip discomfort, and postural problems we will discuss as part of the "Sitting Disease" in Chapter 6.

The Fascial Web

Beneath your skin, surrounding and interweaving through your muscles, bones, nerves, and organs, is a remarkable network of connective tissue called fascia. Imagine a silvery-white, three-dimensional web or bodystocking that connects everything to everything else.

Fascia is not just passive packing material. It helps transmit forces, provides support, allows tissues to glide smoothly over one another, and even plays a role in sensory feedback. Healthy fascia is well-hydrated, pliable, and resilient. However, lack of movement, static postures (hello, chair-sitting!), injury, or inflammation can cause fascia to become dehydrated, stiff, and restricted, sometimes forming adhesions or "sticky spots" between layers that should glide freely.

Movement, especially varied movement that takes joints through large ranges of motion like squatting, is crucial for maintaining healthy fascia. It helps to "wring out" old fluid and allows fresh hydration in, breaks down minor adhesions, and encourages pliability. Think of it as maintaining a well-lubricated, adaptable internal framework. Static sitting does the opposite, potentially contributing to feelings of stiffness and restricted movement not just in muscles, but in this vital connective tissue web as well.

Understanding Your Pelvic Floor

Now, let's talk about a group of muscles often misunderstood or ignored, yet fundamental to core stability, continence, sexual function, and even breathing: the pelvic floor.

What is it? Imagine a broad sling or hammock of muscles stretching from your pubic bone at the front to your tailbone at the back, and spanning side-to-side between your Ischial tuberosities, the bones you sit on. These muscles support your pelvic organs (bladder, uterus/prostate, rectum) and control the openings for urination and defecation.

The Squat Connection: The pelvic floor does not exist in isolation; it works intimately with your diaphragm and deep abdominal muscles as part of that "core canister." Here is the magic of the squat:

As you lower into a deep squat, your pelvic floor muscles naturally lengthen under the load of your descending organs, acting like an elastic brake (an eccentric contraction).

As you rise from the squat, these muscles naturally contract and lift slightly (a concentric contraction), contributing to core stability and assisting the hip extensors. This dynamic lengthening and contracting through a full range is precisely how muscles maintain optimal tone – meaning they are strong, responsive, and flexible. A healthy pelvic floor is not rock hard; it is adaptable.

The Chair Disconnect: Chronic chair-sitting often disconnects us from our pelvic floor. Poor, slumped posture can put downward pressure on these muscles, potentially leading to weakness over time. Alternatively, some people adopt compensatory tension patterns, constantly gripping their pelvic floor or glutes while sitting, leading to tightness, pain, and dysfunction. Neither chronic slackness nor chronic tension is healthy. Furthermore, sitting limits the pelvic floor's ability to move dynamically with the breath and in coordination with the rest of the core. Issues like stress incontinence (leaking with cough/sneeze/laugh), pelvic pain, or feelings of pressure can sometimes be linked back to pelvic floor dysfunction exacerbated by sedentary habits.

Link to Birth (Foreshadowing): As we will explore more in Chapter 8, the ability of the pelvic floor muscles to lengthen and yield appropriately is paramount during childbirth. Practicing deep squats can help cultivate this necessary elasticity and body awareness.

Restoring Elastic Balance

The beauty of the squat lies in its ability to restore balance to this entire system of muscles and fascia. It is not just an exercise to strengthen your legs; it is a fundamental human movement pattern that:

- Activates and strengthens muscles often weakened by sitting (glutes, core).
- Lengthens muscles often shortened by sitting (hip flexors, calves).
- Mobilizes fascia, promoting hydration and gliding.
- Trains the pelvic floor to be both strong and supple through its full dynamic range.
- Enhances body awareness (proprioception) and coordination.
- It encourages your body to function as the integrated, elastic system was designed to be.

Listen to Your Elastic Body

As you begin (or continue) to explore squatting (following the guidance in Chapter 9), pay attention to these elastic tissues. Where do you feel effort? Where do you feel stretch? Where do you feel restriction? Learning to squat well is not just about achieving depth; it is about developing a conversation with your muscles and fascia, understanding where imbalances lie, and patiently working to restore harmony.

Our muscles and connective tissues provide the power, flexibility, and support that allow our skeletal structure (Chapter 4) to move through the world. When we honor their need for dynamic movement like squatting, we foster resilience and health. When we subject them to prolonged static postures like chair-sitting, we invite imbalance and dysfunction. In the next chapter, we will face the consequences head-on, examining the collection of issues often termed the "Sitting Disease."

There Are No Cave Drawings of Chairs

The Dis-ease Of Sitting

"The chair promises comfort but often delivers dysfunction. Our bodies were not built for constant passive support."

Let's be honest. As you read this, where are you? If you are like many people living here in the mid-2020s, chances are you might be sitting. Perhaps in an office chair, a car seat, a comfortable armchair at home, or even on a bus or train. We explored how we arrived at this chair-centric existence in Chapter 3, tracing the rise of seating furniture. And in Chapters 4 and 5, we delved into the amazing way our skeleton and muscles are designed for dynamic movement, including the deep squat.

Now, we must connect those dots and face a somewhat uncomfortable reality: our modern habit of prolonged sitting, hour after hour, day after day, comes at a significant cost to our health.

Researchers and health professionals are increasingly talking about the "Sitting Disease" – not a formal medical diagnosis, but a powerful term capturing the cluster of health problems linked to excessive sedentary behavior, particularly the kind encouraged by chairs. It is the predictable fallout from forcing bodies designed for movement into prolonged static postures. This chapter unpacks some of the most common ways chairs can undermine our well-being, from our aching backs right down to our digestive system.

The Spine's Distress Signal

Low back pain is one of the most common reasons people seek help from chiropractors like me, or from other healthcare providers. Neck pain runs a close second. While many factors can contribute, our sitting habits are often a major culprit. Here is why:

The Dreaded "C-Slump": Remember those natural curves of the spine we discussed in Chapter 4? Especially the inward curve (lordosis) in the lower back? When we collapse into a typical chair slouch, our pelvis tilts backward, and that vital lumbar curve often reverses. We adopt a 'C' shape instead. This posture dramatically increases the pressure on the vertebral discs – the shock absorbers between our spinal bones. Think of squeezing a jelly donut unevenly; the filling bulges out. Prolonged pressure can contribute to disc degeneration, bulging, or even herniation over time, potentially leading to pain, sciatica, or numbness/tingling down the legs.

There Are No Cave Drawings of Chairs

Core Deactivation: As we learned in Chapter 5, sitting passively tells our deep core muscles – the abdominal wall, back extensors, pelvic floor, diaphragm – that they can switch off. Without this active muscular "corset" stabilizing the spine, the load falls more heavily on the passive structures like discs and ligaments, making them more vulnerable to strain and injury.

"Text Neck" and Forward Head Posture: When sitting at desks, looking at computer screens, or hunching over smartphones (often done while sitting!), we tend to jut our heads forward. For every inch your head moves forward from its optimal alignment over your shoulders, its effective weight on your neck and upper back muscles increase significantly. Imagine holding a bowling ball close to your body versus holding it out at arm's length – the strain is much greater further away. This chronic strain contributes to neck pain, shoulder tension, upper back aches, and even tension headaches.

For many people struggling with chronic back and neck pain, reducing prolonged static sitting and incorporating more movement (including postures like squatting that encourage better alignment) can be a crucial part of finding relief.

Hip Hijinks: The Tightness/Weakness Trap

Our hips, those amazing ball-and-socket joints built for mobility (Chapter 4), also suffer significantly from chair dependence:

Locked Short: *The Hip Flexor Problem*: Sitting keeps your hips in a state of flexion (bent). The muscles at the front of your hips, the hip flexors, adapt to this by becoming chronically shortened and tight (as mentioned in Chapter 5). Tight hip flexors can pull the pelvis forward into an anterior tilt, which can, in turn, increase the arch in the lower back and contribute to low back pain. They can also restrict hip extension – the ability to fully straighten your hip – which is vital for walking, running, and simply standing upright efficiently.

Switched Off: *Gluteal Amnesia*: While your hip flexors are getting tight, your powerful gluteal muscles (buttocks) are getting sleepy. Sitting on them for hours sends a clear signal: "You are not needed right now." Over time, they can become weak and develop poor firing patterns – they essentially "forget" how to activate properly when you do need them (like when standing up or climbing stairs). This "gluteal amnesia" forces other muscles, like hamstrings or lower back muscles, to compensate, leading to strain, fatigue, and potential injury in those areas.

Stiff Joints: Without regularly moving through their full range (like in a squat), the hip joints themselves can become stiff. The joint capsule can tighten, and the cartilage may not receive the nourishment it needs (Chapter 4), potentially contributing to conditions like osteoarthritis later in life.

This combination of tight hip flexors and weak glutes is an incredibly common pattern in sedentary populations and is a major driver of movement dysfunction and pain.

Knees, Shoulders, and Beyond

While the spine and hips bear the brunt, the negative effects of poor sitting posture can ripple outwards. Altered forces due to pelvic tilt and weak glutes can contribute to knee pain. Slumped posture often leads to rounded shoulders and tightness in the chest muscles. Even prolonged poor positioning at a desk can contribute to wrist and elbow problems like carpal tunnel syndrome or tennis elbow, although these are more related to specific ergonomics than sitting itself. The point is, the body functions as an interconnected system; dysfunction in one area often creates compensation and stress elsewhere.

Beyond Aches/Pains

The consequences of excessive sitting extend beyond the musculoskeletal system. Our metabolism and circulation also take a hit:

Metabolic Slump: Large muscles, particularly those in the legs and buttocks, play a significant role in regulating blood sugar and burning fat. When these muscles are inactive for long periods while sitting, your body's ability to manage blood sugar effectively decreases, and your overall metabolic rate slows down. Research increasingly links high amounts of sedentary time (independent of exercise time) to an increased risk of developing metabolic syndrome (a cluster of conditions including high blood pressure, high blood sugar, unhealthy cholesterol levels, and abdominal fat), type 2 diabetes, and cardiovascular disease.

Stagnant Circulation: Sitting for hours can impede blood flow, especially in the lower legs. Gravity causes blood to pool, increasing pressure in the veins. This can contribute to swollen ankles, varicose veins, and, in rare but serious cases of prolonged immobility (like long flights), increase the risk of deep vein thrombosis (DVT), a blood clot in the leg veins. Reduced circulation also means less efficient delivery of oxygen and nutrients to tissues and slower removal of waste products.

Dr. Chada

This highlights a critical point: even if you meet recommended exercise guidelines, spending the rest of your day largely sedentary can still pose significant health risks.

The Gut Suffers

Your digestive system is not immune to the effects of sitting either:

Compression: Slouching can physically compress your abdominal cavity, potentially putting pressure on your digestive organs and hindering their optimal function.

Slowed Motility?: While research is ongoing, some experts suggest that lack of movement might contribute to slower bowel motility (the movement of waste through your intestines).

The Toilet Trouble: As discussed previously (Chapter 3 and 5), the seated position on a typical Western toilet is biomechanically less efficient for defecation than squatting. It requires more straining, which can contribute to constipation, hemorrhoids, and potentially even diverticulosis over the long term. Chronic constipation itself can lead to discomfort, bloating, and other issues.

Overlooked Issues: The Pelvic Floor Under Pressure

The pelvic floor muscles, that crucial hammock at the base of our core (Chapter 5), are particularly vulnerable to the effects of poor sitting posture:

There Are No Cave Drawings of Chairs

Chronic Pressure or Slackness: Slumping can place sustained downward pressure on the pelvic floor. Alternatively, a lack of engagement can lead to weakness.

Excessive Tension: Some people compensate for poor core stability by habitually clenching their glutes or pelvic floor while sitting, leading to muscle tightness, trigger points, and pelvic pain.

Functional Consequences: Pelvic floor dysfunction can manifest as stress urinary incontinence (leaking urine when coughing, sneezing, or laughing), fecal incontinence, pelvic organ prolapse (where organs descend due to lack of support), and chronic pelvic pain syndromes. While multiple factors contribute to these conditions, poor posture and sedentary habits are increasingly recognized as significant contributors or exacerbating factors.

Losing Your Functional Freedom

Perhaps one of the most insidious effects of chronic chair-sitting is the gradual erosion of our overall functional mobility. Our bodies adhere strictly to the "use it or lose it" principle (Chapter 4). If you consistently avoid moving into deep squats, bending fully at the hips, or reaching overhead, your body adapts by restricting those movements.

You might first notice it as increased stiffness when trying to get up from the floor. Then maybe difficulty bending down to tie your shoes or pick something up. Over time, this loss of functional range can impact your ability to participate fully in life, increase your risk of falls, and contribute to a sense of physical frailty. Sitting essentially trains your body to become very good at sitting, but progressively less capable at almost everything else.

You Cannot Out-Exercise Excessive Sitting

This is a vital takeaway. Many people believe that hitting the gym for an hour a few times a week compensates for sitting 8, 10, or even 12 hours a day. Unfortunately, research suggests otherwise. While exercise is incredibly important, it does not fully negate the risks associated with prolonged sedentary time. Think of it like smoking – going for a run does not cancel out the damage from cigarettes. Similarly, your workout does not entirely undo the metabolic and postural effects of sitting the vast majority of your remaining hours. Reducing total sitting time and breaking it up frequently is just as important, if not more so, than dedicated exercise sessions.

Recognize Yourself? There is Hope!

As you read through this list of potential problems, you might be nodding along, recognizing some of these aches, pains, or limitations in your own body or in those around you. Please do no feel discouraged or blamed. Our modern environment, as we saw in Chapter 3, strongly encourages these sedentary habits. The goal here is to understand. Recognizing why these issues might be occurring – seeing the connection between our chairs and our health challenges – is the crucial first step toward making positive changes.

The good news is that our bodies are remarkably adaptable in a positive direction too! By understanding the detrimental effects of excessive sitting, we empower ourselves to counteract them.

In the next chapter, we will finally shift our focus fully to the positive side – exploring the wide-ranging benefits you can gain by reducing chair time and intentionally reintroducing more natural postures, especially the fundamental squat, back into your life. The Dis-ease of sitting is prevalent, but it is not an inevitable sentence.

There Are No Cave Drawings of Chairs

Reclaiming Your Natural Nature

"We often forget the primal... consider that most of us were probably conceived by at least one person in a squatted position."

Reading the last chapter might have felt a bit heavy. Confronting the potential health consequences of our modern sitting habits – the back pain, the stiffness, the metabolic slowdown, what researchers call the "Sitting Disease" – can be discouraging, especially when chairs seem so unavoidable. But here is the wonderful, empowering truth: Your body is incredibly resilient and inherently designed for health and movement. While chronic sitting can lead us down a path of dysfunction, embracing more natural postures, especially the fundamental squat, offers a powerful way back towards reclaiming your body's natural blueprint for vitality.

Think of it like rediscovering a language your body used to know fluently (way back in toddlerhood, as we saw in Chapter 1, or ancestrally, as explored in Chapter 2). Relearning to squat is not about forcing your body into some new, stressful position; it is about reawakening its innate capabilities. The benefits ripple outwards, touching nearly every aspect of your physical well-being. Let's explore some of the most significant rewards you can gain by inviting the squat back into your life.

Freedom Through Mobility

Remember how we discussed joints needing their "motion is lotion" (Chapter 4)? Squatting is perhaps the most efficient way to provide this for your entire lower body simultaneously.

Happy Hips: The deep flexion involved helps maintain or restore mobility in those crucial ball-and-socket joints, counteracting the stiffness often caused by sitting (Chapter 6). This means easier bending, less potential pinching, and greater overall freedom in hip movement.

Nourished Knees: Taking your knees through their full, natural range of motion during a squat helps circulate synovial fluid, nourishing the cartilage and keeping the joint healthy. It reminds the knee joint of its full potential beyond that static 90-degree chair angle.

Agile Ankles: Regularly asking your ankles to dorsiflex (bend deeply) as you squat helps maintain the flexibility needed not just for squatting, but for walking, climbing stairs, and preventing compensations that can lead to knee or back pain (Chapter 4).

Consistently incorporating squats can lead to a noticeable decrease in joint stiffness and an increase in your overall sense of fluid, easy movement.

There Are No Cave Drawings of Chairs

Building Real-World Strength

Squatting is not just a "leg exercise"; it is a fundamental human movement that builds practical, functional strength like few other activities can.

Integrated Power: Squats engage multiple large muscle groups – quadriceps, glutes, hamstrings, calves, and the entire core canister (Chapter 5) – all working together in coordination. This builds strength that translates directly to real-world activities far better than isolated exercises on machines might.

Waking Up the Glutes: By taking the hips through a large range of motion and requiring powerful extension to stand up, squats are fantastic for combating "gluteal amnesia" (Chapter 6). Strong, active glutes are essential for hip health, athletic movement, and crucially, for protecting your lower back by preventing compensatory strain.

Core Stability: A well-executed squat demands and develops core stiffness – that coordinated bracing action involving your deep abdominals, back muscles, diaphragm, and pelvic floor (Chapter 5). This stability protects your spine not just during the squat, but during lifting, carrying, pushing, or pulling activities in daily life.

The strength gained from squatting makes everyday tasks – carrying groceries, lifting children, getting up from a low seat (or the floor!), gardening, engaging in sports – feel easier and safer.

Standing Taller: Improving Your Posture Naturally

Tired of slouching? Squatting can indirectly, yet powerfully, improve your standing and moving posture.

Stronger Foundation: By strengthening the glutes and core muscles responsible for holding your pelvis and spine in optimal alignment, squatting provides the necessary muscular support for better posture.

Increased Awareness: The process of learning to squat correctly (which we will cover in Chapter 9) inherently increases your body awareness (proprioception). You become more attuned to your spinal position, pelvic tilt, and muscle engagement, and this awareness carries over into how you sit, stand, and move throughout the day.

Counteracting the Slump: Improving hip flexor length and thoracic (mid-back) mobility, both benefits of good squatting, helps counteract the hunched, C-slump posture bred by chair-sitting (Chapter 6).

Better posture is not just about looking more confident; it is about reducing strain on your joints and muscles, allowing your body to function more efficiently.

Easing Common Aches and Pains

For many people plagued by the chronic aches discussed in Chapter 6, incorporating appropriate squatting can be a game-changer:

Soothing Your Back: By strengthening core support, activating the glutes (taking the load off the back), improving hip mobility, and decompressing spinal discs relative to prolonged sitting, squatting can significantly reduce or even eliminate low back pain for many individuals.

There Are No Cave Drawings of Chairs

Freeing Your Hips: Restoring range of motion and balancing muscle activation around the hip can alleviate stiffness and pain often associated with tight hip flexors or the early stages of arthritis.

Comforting Your Knees: Improved cartilage health, stronger supporting muscles (quads, hamstrings, glutes), and better movement patterns due to improved hip and ankle mobility can often lead to a noticeable reduction in knee pain. (Caveat: requires proper form and addressing underlying issues).

Of course, if you have significant pain, seeking professional guidance (like from a chiropractor or physical therapist) is essential, but squatting, done correctly, is often a key part of the solution.

Optimizing Digestion and Elimination

This might seem surprising, but squatting can significantly benefit your digestive health:

Nature's Angle for Elimination: As we have touched upon (Chapters 3, 5, 6), the squatting posture naturally aligns the rectum and relaxes the puborectalis muscle, allowing for easier, faster, and more complete bowel movements. This can help prevent straining, reduce constipation, and lower the risk of developing hemorrhoids or potentially aggravating conditions like diverticulosis. It is simply working with your body's plumbing design.

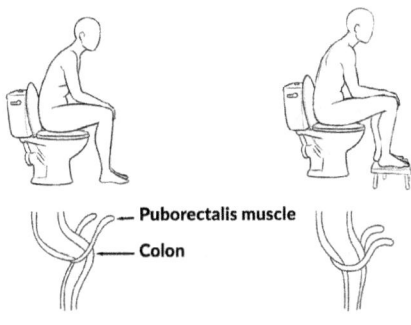

Gentle Internal Massage?: While less direct, the deep folding action of a squat might provide a gentle compressive massage to the abdominal organs, potentially stimulating movement within the digestive tract (peristalsis).

For overall gut health and comfort, adopting a squatting position for elimination (using a Squatty Potty® or similar device if needed) can make a world of difference.

Pelvic Floor Health

The dynamic nature of the squat offers unique benefits for the often-neglected pelvic floor muscles (Chapter 5):

Optimal Tone: Unlike sitting which can lead to weakness or excessive tension (Chapter 6), squatting encourages the pelvic floor to work through its full range – lengthening eccentrically on the way down, contracting concentrically on the way up. This builds responsive strength and flexibility.

Improved Coordination: Squatting helps integrate the pelvic floor with the breath and the rest of the deep core muscles, improving overall coordination and stability.

Support and Continence: A well-toned, coordinated pelvic floor provides better support for pelvic organs and improves bladder and bowel control, potentially reducing issues like stress incontinence. This is relevant for both women and men at all stages of life.

Birth Preparation: As we will explore specifically in Chapter 8, the elasticity and strength developed through squatting can be highly beneficial during labor and delivery.

There Are No Cave Drawings of Chairs

Better Balance and Stability

Worried about falls, especially as you get older? Squatting is excellent balance training. It requires your nervous system to coordinate muscle actions across your feet, ankles, knees, and hips to keep you stable. Strengthening these stabilizing muscles and improving joint mobility directly translates to better balance during walking and other activities, reducing the risk of potentially devastating falls.

A Circulation Boost

Remember how sitting can cause blood to pool in the legs (Chapter 6)? Activating the large muscles of your legs during squats acts like a powerful pump, helping to push blood back up towards your heart. This improves circulation, delivering fresh oxygen to tissues and helping to flush out metabolic waste products.

Freedom in Intimacy

While not often discussed, the physical benefits of squatting can extend to sexual health and comfort. Improved hip mobility allows for a greater range of motion and potentially more comfortable positioning. Enhanced core strength and pelvic floor awareness and tone can also contribute positively to sexual function and sensation for both partners. It is another way of reclaiming your body's natural movement freedom.

The Big Picture

Ultimately, the benefits of squatting add up to something profound: an increase in your overall functional capacity and vitality. It is about more than just isolated improvements; it is about maintaining the physical ability to engage fully and freely with the world around you.

Being able to squat comfortably means you can more easily get up and down from the floor, pick things up without straining your back, play with children or pets at their level, navigate uneven terrain, and generally move through life with greater ease, confidence, and resilience. It connects you back to the physical competence that was the birthright of our ancestors (Chapter 2) and helps you resist the physical decline so often accelerated by sedentary modern life.

Ready to Begin?

The case for the squat is compelling. It is a fundamental human movement packed with benefits that directly counteract the harms of excessive sitting. It nurtures our joints, builds functional strength, improves posture, aids digestion, supports our core, enhances balance, and boosts overall vitality. It is a powerful tool for reclaiming your natural blueprint.

Now that you understand the why – the history, the anatomy, the problems of sitting, and the profound benefits of squatting – you might be wondering about the how. How do you safely start incorporating squats if you have not done them in years? How do you work around limitations? Do no worry, Chapter 9 is dedicated entirely to providing a practical, step-by-step guide. But first, in Chapter 8, we will take a focused look at one particularly powerful application of squatting: its remarkable benefits during childbirth.

There Are No Cave Drawings of Chairs

Primal Birth as Nature Intended

"The pelvis is designed to open; our chosen birth positions should allow it, not restrict it."

Throughout this book, we have explored how reconnecting with fundamental human movements, particularly the squat, aligns with our body's inherent design, offering benefits from joint health (Chapter 4) to core stability and pelvic floor function (Chapter 5 & 7). Now, we turn to perhaps the most primal and powerful event for which the female body is designed: giving birth. Just as our ancestors squatted to rest and work (Chapter 2), historical and cross-cultural evidence suggests that upright, mobile positions, including squatting, were once common, intuitive postures for labor and delivery.

In stark contrast, the image most associated with birth in modern Western culture is often a woman lying on her back in a hospital bed (the lithotomy or semi-reclined position). While medical interventions and specific circumstances sometimes necessitate particular positions, this chapter explores the compelling biomechanical and physiological reasons why embracing gravity and mobility through squatting and other primal postures can often facilitate a more efficient, empowering, and potentially safer birth experience, working with the body's incredible innate wisdom. This information is offered to help expecting parents and those supporting them understand the possibilities and make informed choices.

The Adaptable Pelvis

First, let's appreciate the brilliance of the female pelvis. As we touched on in Chapter 4, the pelvis is not one solid bone. It is composed of several bones connected by joints – notably the sacroiliac joints at the back (connecting the sacrum to the iliac bones) and the pubic symphysis at the front. During pregnancy, hormones like relaxin soften the ligaments around these joints, allowing for increased flexibility and movement. This is not a design flaw; it is a feature! It allows the pelvis to subtly shift and expand during labor to make space for the baby's passage. The key, however, is being in a position that allows this natural adaptability to occur.

How Squatting Maximizes Pelvic Space

This is where birthing position becomes critical. The dimensions of the pelvic outlet – the bony opening at the bottom of the pelvis that the baby must navigate – can change significantly depending on the mother's posture.

There Are No Cave Drawings of Chairs

The Restriction of Lying Down: When a birthing person lies on their back or in a semi-reclined position (common in many hospital settings), their sacrum (the triangular bone at the base of the spine) and coccyx (tailbone) are pressed against the bed or mattress. This immobilizes the back of the pelvis, preventing the tailbone from moving freely out of the way and potentially decreasing the front-to-back diameter of the outlet. The weight bearing down on the sacrum can also limit the natural widening of the ischial tuberosities (bones you sit on).

The Advantage of Squatting: In contrast, a deep squat (whether supported or unsupported) allows amazing things to happen:

The femurs (thigh bones) press outwards, encouraging the ischial tuberosities to widen, increasing the side-to-side diameter of the outlet.

Crucially, the sacrum and tailbone are free to move backward, significantly increasing the front-to-back diameter. Imagine trying to get a large piece of furniture through a doorway – you'd open the door as wide as possible, right? Squatting essentially opens the pelvic "door" to its maximum potential. Studies have shown that the pelvic outlet area can increase by as much as 25-30% in a squatting position compared to lying down! That extra space can make a crucial difference for the baby's descent and rotation.

Letting Gravity Lend a Hand

This benefit is beautifully simple: physics works! When the birthing person is in an upright position – squatting, kneeling, standing, leaning – gravity naturally assists the baby's downward movement through the birth canal. Contractions work with gravity to encourage descent. When lying on the back, contractions must work against gravity, potentially leading to slower progress or the need for more forceful pushing. Utilizing gravity is one of the most intuitive ways to support the physiological process of labor.

Working Smarter: Uterine Efficiency

There is evidence to suggest that upright positions may also lead to more efficient and effective uterine contractions. Why?

Better Alignment: Upright postures can help the baby align optimally within the pelvis, ensuring the pressure from the baby's head is applied evenly to the cervix, which can stimulate stronger, more coordinated contractions.

Improved Blood Flow: Lying flat on the back can potentially compress major blood vessels (the aorta and vena cava) running behind the uterus, potentially reducing blood flow to both the uterus and the baby. Upright positions avoid this compression, potentially allowing the uterine muscles to function more effectively. Some studies suggest labor may progress more quickly in upright, mobile positions compared to recumbent ones.

Protecting the Perineum

The perineum is the area of tissue between the vaginal opening and the anus. Tearing of this tissue during delivery is common, but the severity can vary. Squatting may help minimize significant tearing:

Even Pressure: In a squat, as the baby's head crowns, the perineal tissues tend to stretch more evenly and gradually compared to the focused pressure often experienced when lying on the back with legs pulled up (lithotomy).

There Are No Cave Drawings of Chairs

Relaxation: Squatting can encourage relaxation of the pelvic floor muscles (as they reach their lengthened state - Chapter 5), allowing for a gentler yielding of the tissues.

Reduced Need for Episiotomy: When tissues stretch more effectively, there may be less perceived need for an episiotomy (a surgical cut to enlarge the vaginal opening), which carries its own risks.

Baby's Journey: Optimal Positioning and Oxygen

The baby is an active participant in birth! Position matters for them too.

Fetal Positioning: Upright positions and movement can encourage the baby to settle into the optimal Occiput Anterior (OA) position (facing the mother's back), which generally makes for an easier passage through the pelvis. Positions like hands-and-knees are particularly helpful for rotating a baby from a posterior ("back labor") position.

Oxygen Supply: As mentioned regarding blood flow, avoiding compression of major blood vessels by staying upright may contribute to a more stable oxygen supply for the baby throughout labor.

A Family of Primal Positions

While squatting is powerful, it is not the only beneficial "primal" position. Freedom of movement is key! Other excellent options include:

Hands-and-Knees: Fantastic for relieving back pain during labor ("back labor"), allows the belly to hang freely, uses gravity, promotes pelvic mobility, and aids fetal rotation.

Kneeling (Upright or Leaning Forward): Uses gravity, allows pelvic movement, takes pressure off the back. Leaning forward over a birth ball, bed, or partner can feel very supportive.

Standing/Walking/Leaning: Utilizes gravity, encourages descent, allowing for swaying or rocking motions which can ease pain and help labor progress.

Side-Lying: A good resting position that still avoids vena cava compression and allows for some pelvic mobility (especially if the upper leg is supported).

The common thread? They avoid the restrictions of lying flat on the back and allow the birthing person to move intuitively and work with their body and gravity.

A Brief Look Back

If upright positions offer so many advantages, how did lying down become the standard in many Western settings? Historically, women birthed in positions they found most comfortable, often upright or kneeling, attended by midwives (as briefly mentioned in Chapter 3). The shift towards hospital births and physician-led care in the 19th and 20th centuries brought changes:

Physician Convenience: The lithotomy position provides easier visual and physical access for the attending physician, especially for monitoring and interventions.

There Are No Cave Drawings of Chairs

Anesthesia: The introduction of epidurals often necessitates more restricted positions due to loss of sensation and motor control in the lower body (though not always complete immobility).

Cultural Factors: Birth became increasingly medicalized, sometimes prioritizing technological monitoring and intervention over physiological processes and maternal intuition.

While medical observation and intervention are sometimes crucial, routinely placing low-risk birthing individuals in positions known to be biomechanically suboptimal warrants questioning.

Empowerment Through Knowledge and Choice

Understanding the biomechanics of birth positions empowers expecting parents. It allows you to:

Have Informed Discussions: Talk to your midwife or doctor about your preferences for movement and positioning during labor before the event. Ask about their typical practices and hospital policies.

Create a Birth Plan: Include your preferences for positioning and freedom of movement.

Consider Your Birth Environment: Choose a setting (hospital, birth center, home) and care providers who are supportive of physiological birth and movement.

Seek Support: Consider hiring a doula, who can provide continuous physical and emotional support and help advocate for your preferences, including position changes.

Connecting Birth Positions to Your Squatting Journey

The ability to comfortably get into and hold a squat or other deep knee/hip bending positions can make utilizing these beneficial postures during labor much easier. The pelvic floor awareness, core connection, and hip mobility cultivated through practicing squats (Chapters 5 & 7, and the 'how-to' in Chapter 9) can directly prepare your body for the physical demands of labor and delivery.

Trusting the Body's Design

Childbirth is a powerful, transformative event. By understanding and respecting the body's inherent biomechanical design, we can create conditions that favor a more physiological process. Utilizing gravity, maximizing pelvic dimensions through positions like squatting or hands-and-knees, and allowing freedom of movement are not radical ideas; they are rooted in ancient wisdom and supported by modern anatomical understanding. While every birth journey is unique, embracing these primal postures offers a pathway to potentially enhance comfort, efficiency, and empowerment during this incredible rite of passage.

Now that we have explored this specific, powerful application, let's broaden our focus again. In the next chapter, we will get down to the practicalities: how can anyone safely and effectively start incorporating the squat back into their daily life to reap the many benefits we have discussed?

There Are No Cave Drawings of Chairs

A Practical Guide to Reclaiming the Squat

"Reclaiming movement is not about force; it is about listening, preparing, and progressing patiently. Your body remembers."

We have journeyed through history (Chapters 2 & 3), explored the intricate design of our bodies (Chapters 4 & 5), faced the potential consequences of our modern sitting habits (Chapter 6), and celebrated the profound benefits of reclaiming natural movement (Chapter 7), including its power in childbirth (Chapter 8). By now, I hope you are convinced that the squat is not just some arbitrary exercise, but a fundamental human posture with incredible potential for improving your health and vitality.

The big question remaining is likely: "Okay, I am inspired... but how do I actually start? Especially if the idea of doing a deep squat right now feels like climbing Mount Everest?"

This chapter is your practical roadmap. It is designed to guide you, step-by-step, on a journey to safely and effectively reintroducing squatting into your life. Forget images of super-flexible yogis or elite athletes; this is about meeting your body where it is right now, here on _____ (fill in today's date) and patiently working towards greater freedom and function. Remember, this is a process of rediscovery, not a race. Progress, not perfection, is the goal.

Step 1: Know Your Starting Point (A Quick Self-Assessment)

Before diving into squatting itself, let's get a sense of your current mobility in the key areas required (as we discussed anatomically in Chapter 4). These simple checks are not tests to pass or fail; they are just information gatherings to help guide your preparation. Perform these gently.

Ankle Check (Dorsiflexion): Stand facing a wall with your shoes off. Place one foot straight forward, big toe just a few inches from the wall. Keeping your heel flat on the floor, bend your knee straight forward, trying to touch the wall. If you can touch the wall easily, move your foot back slightly and try again. Find the furthest distance your big toe can be from the wall while still allowing your knee to touch without your heel lifting. Good mobility is generally considered around 4-5 inches. Less than that suggests your ankles might be limiting your squat depth. Repeat on the other side.

There Are No Cave Drawings of Chairs

Hip Check (Flexion): Lie flat on your back with both legs straight. Gently pull one knee towards your chest, holding behind the thigh or below the kneecap. Keep your other leg flat on the floor (do no let it lift). How far does your knee come towards your chest? Do you feel any pinching or blocking sensation in the front of the hip? Ideally, the thigh should come close to the chest without pain. Compare sides.

Movement Pattern Check (Optional Bodyweight Squat): Stand with your feet about shoulder-width apart, toes pointing slightly outwards. Raise your arms straight out in front of you for balance. Slowly lower yourself into a squat, going only as low as you comfortably can while maintaining good form. Pay attention:

- Do your heels lift off the ground? (Suggests ankle restriction)
- Does your lower back round significantly? (Suggests hip mobility or core control issues)
- Do your knees cave inwards? (Suggests hip/glute weakness or ankle issues)
- Do you lean excessively far forward? (Often compensates for ankle/hip restriction)

Dr. Chada

Again, this is just information. If you notice restrictions, that is okay! It simply highlights where the preparatory work in Step 2 will be most beneficial.

Step 2: Prepare the Ground (Mobilizations & Stretches)

Just like you would not start gardening without preparing the soil, it is wise to prepare your joints and tissues before asking them to squat deeply. Incorporate these gentle movements regularly, especially before practicing your squats. Listen to your body and only move within a pain-free range.

For Your Ankles (Improve Dorsiflexion):

Calf Stretches: Stand facing a wall, step one foot back, keeping the back knee straight and heel down for the gastrocnemius stretch (hold 30s). Then, slightly bend the back knee, keeping the heel down, for the soleus stretch (hold 30s). Repeat on the other side.

There Are No Cave Drawings of Chairs

Ankle Circles: Sit or stand, lift one foot slightly, and slowly draw circles with your big toe, moving only at the ankle. Go clockwise and counter-clockwise.

For Your Hips (Improve Flexion & Rotation):

Kneeling Hip Flexor Stretch: Kneel on one knee (use padding if needed), place the other foot flat on the floor in front. Gently tuck your tailbone slightly and shift your weight forward until you feel a stretch in the front of the hip of the kneeling leg. Hold 30s. Repeat on other side.

90/90 Stretch: Sit on the floor. Bend one leg in front of you with the knee at roughly 90 degrees. Bend the other leg behind you, also aiming for 90 degrees at the knee. Try to sit upright. You should feel a stretch in the hip/glute of the front leg and potentially the front of the hip of the back leg. Hold 30-60s. Switch sides. (Modify if painful).

Dr. Chada

For Your Spine (Gentle Movement):

Cat-Cow: Start on your hands and knees. As you inhale, gently arch your back, dropping your belly and looking slightly up (*Cow*). As you exhale, round your spine towards the ceiling, tucking your chin and tailbone (*Cat*). Move slowly and smoothly for 5-10 breaths.

Step 3: Relearning the Movement (Squat Progressions)

Now, let's start squatting! The key is to begin where you feel stable and successful, focusing on good form, and gradually progressing the depth and reducing the support. Maintain these cues throughout: Keep heels grounded. Keep chest relatively lifted (avoid excessive rounding of the back). Allow knees to track generally over your second or third toes (do no let them collapse inward).

Supported Squat: Stand facing a sturdy kitchen counter, table edge, door frame handles, or use a suspension trainer (like TRX straps) if available. Hold on lightly for balance and support. Place

There Are No Cave Drawings of Chairs

feet shoulder-width apart (or slightly wider), toes slightly out. Initiate the movement by sending your hips back slightly, then bend your knees, lowering yourself as far as comfortable while maintaining form and keeping heels down. Use your arms minimally for support, primarily for balance. Pause briefly, then drive through your heels to stand back up. Start with 5-10 repetitions.

Box Squat: Place a sturdy chair, bench, low stool, or stack of stable books behind you. Stand in front of it, feet in your squat stance. Perform a squat as above, lowering yourself until your buttocks lightly touch the object behind you. Do no crash down or fully sit and relax. Tap lightly, then immediately stand back up, squeezing your glutes at the top. This builds control and confidence with depth. As you get stronger and more mobile, gradually use a lower object. Aim for 8-12 repetitions.

Assisted Deep Squat: If balance or achieving depth is still tricky, try holding a light weight (5-10 lbs. dumbbell, kettlebell, even a heavy book) out in front of your chest (a "Goblet Squat").

This counterweight often makes it easier to sit back and keep your balance as you go deeper. Alternatively, you can lightly hold onto a stable pole or door frame for balance assistance, especially at the very bottom of the squat. Focus on feeling the stretch and position.

Unassisted Bodyweight Squat: Once you feel comfortable with the above, progress to squatting using only your bodyweight. Focus on smooth, controlled movement down and up. Aim for a depth where your hips are at least parallel to your knees, or deeper if comfortable and form allows. Work towards 10-15 repetitions.

Deep Resting Squat (The Goal Posture): This is the passive, relaxed squat we discussed as an ancestral resting posture (Chapter 2). It often takes time to achieve comfortably. You might need to start by elevating your heels slightly on a rolled towel or thin book. Let your elbows rest inside or outside your knees. Try to relax your back and hips. Hold initially for just 15-30 seconds, gradually increasing the duration as comfort allows. This is not about reps but about reclaiming this as a comfortable resting position.

Step 4: Weave it Into Your Day (Daily Integration)

Practicing squat progressions is great, but the real magic happens when you start integrating more squatting and less sitting into your everyday life:

Movement Snacks: Set a timer to get up from your chair every 30-60 minutes. Do a few gentle squats (supported if needed), some ankle circles, or a Cat-Cow stretch. Break up prolonged sitting!

Embrace Floor Time: When relaxing at home, try spending some time on the floor instead of the sofa. Start with comfortable positions like sitting cross-legged, side-sitting, or kneeling. Gradually experiment with short periods in a supported resting squat.

Bathroom Biomechanics: Use a footstool (like a Squatty Potty® or even sturdy blocks) to elevate your feet when using the toilet. This mimics a more squat-like angle, aiding elimination (as discussed in Chapter 7).

Low-Level Tasks: When picking up light objects, consciously practice using a squat pattern instead of bending only at the waist. Keep your back straight, bend your knees and hips. (Use proper lifting mechanics for heavy items!)

Play at Their Level: If you interact with children or pets, try getting down to their level by squatting or kneeling instead of bending over.

Crucial Considerations: Listen! Prioritize Safety!

This is the most important section. Your body sends signals; learn to listen.

Pain vs. Discomfort: Muscle fatigue, soreness after trying a new movement, or the sensation of tissues stretching is generally okay (discomfort). Sharp, pinching, burning, or deep joint pain is

NOT okay. Pain is your body's stop sign. Do not push through joint pain.

Go Slow and Steady: Be patient! Mobility and strength take time to build, especially if you have been sedentary for years. Consistency is far more important than intensity. Start with easier variations and fewer repetitions, and only progress when you feel ready and pain-free.

Breathe: Do no hold your breath. Try to inhale as you lower (if comfortable) and exhale as you exert effort to stand up or simply breathe naturally throughout.

Modify, Do no Force: If something does not feel right, adjust.

Heels lifting? Temporarily place a thin book or rolled mat under your heels while you continue working on ankle stretches. Gradually reduce the heel lift over time.

Knees caving in? Focus on actively pushing your knees outwards slightly (tracking over your toes). You can practice with a light resistance band around your thighs just above the knees for feedback.

Back rounding excessively? Reduce your squat depth for now. Focus on engaging your core and keeping your chest lifted. Use more support. Work on hip and spine mobility.

When to Seek Professional Help: If you have persistent pain, significant mobility restrictions that do no improve with gentle stretching, or pre-existing joint conditions (like diagnosed arthritis, past surgeries, etc.), it is wise to consult a qualified healthcare professional before starting. A chiropractor, physical therapist, or certified personal trainer with experience in corrective exercise can provide personalized guidance and ensure you are moving safely and effectively.

There Are No Cave Drawings of Chairs
Your Journey Back to Your Foundation

Reclaiming your squat is a journey back to a fundamental part of your human blueprint. It is about restoring movement freedom, building resilience, and enhancing your overall health and well-being. Follow these steps patiently: Assess where you are, prepare your body, progress gradually through the squat variations, Integrate the movement into daily life, and always, always Listen to your body's wisdom.

In the final chapter, we will zoom out one last time, reflecting on this journey and offering some concluding thoughts on how embracing movement beyond the chair can help you reconnect more deeply with your amazing body.

Dr. Chada

Beyond the Chair

"We forget we are mammals and primates before Homo sapiens because we live in captivity."

We began this journey together standing before an imaginary cave wall, puzzled by a simple observation: among the vivid depictions of ancient life, there were no drawings of chairs (Chapter 1). That simple question opened a doorway into exploring our deep human history, revealing a time when resting, working, and living happened largely at ground level, with the squat as a fundamental posture (Chapter 2). We then traced the relatively recent rise of the chair, an invention that gradually reshaped our environment and our habits, leading us away from that ancestral foundation (Chapter 3).

There Are No Cave Drawings of Chairs

Through the lens of anatomy and biomechanics, we uncovered the elegant design of our bodies – skeletons truly built to bend (Chapter 4) and muscles designed for dynamic, elastic strength (Chapter 5). We confronted the uncomfortable truth that our modern, chair-dominated lifestyle often clashes with this design, contributing to a host of issues collectively known as the "Sitting Disease" (Chapter 6).

But crucially, we did not stop there. We celebrated the incredible potential for healing and vitality that comes from reclaiming natural movement, exploring the wide-ranging benefits of the squat – from healthier joints and improved digestion to a more resilient pelvic floor and even potentially smoother childbirth (Chapters 7 & 8). And most recently, we mapped out a practical path, offering assessments, preparations, and progressions to help you safely rediscover the squat and weave more movement back into your daily life (Chapter 9).

Now, as we arrive at the end of this book, let's zoom out one last time. What does all this mean for you, living your life right here, right now, on _____ (fill in today's date)? How can you carry these insights beyond these pages?

The Core Message

If there is one central message, I hope you take away, it is this: Your body possesses innate wisdom and a remarkable capacity for health, vitality, and movement. The aches, pains, stiffness, and limitations many experience in our modern world are often not inevitable consequences of aging, but rather symptoms of a lifestyle that has drifted too far from our biological blueprint – a blueprint designed for dynamic interaction with our environment.

Reclaiming movements like the squat is not about adopting some extreme new fitness regime. It is about honoring that blueprint. It is about giving your joints the varied motion they crave, activating the muscles designed to support you, nourishing your tissues through movement, and ultimately, allowing your body to function more closely to the way it was intended.

Progress, Not Perfection

As you continue applying the practical steps from Chapter 9, please remember to be kind and patient with yourself. If you have spent years primarily sitting, reclaiming mobility and strength will not happen overnight. There will be days when you feel more mobile, and days when you feel stiffer. Some stretches might feel easy, while achieving a deep squat might remain challenging for a while.

That is okay.

The goal is not to achieve a "perfect" Instagram-worthy squat by next Tuesday. The goal is the process – the consistent, mindful effort to move a little more, sit a little less, and listen to your body's feedback. Celebrate small victories: holding a resting squat for 10 seconds longer, noticing less back stiffness after a day of incorporating movement breaks, feeling strong enough to easily pick up a grandchild. It is the gradual accumulation of these small changes that leads to profound shifts in well-being over time.

This is not about adding another stressful "should" to your life. It is about finding joy and freedom in movement, making choices that feel good and nourishing to your body. Think of it as becoming more "chair-conscious" rather than striving to be entirely "chair-less" – making deliberate choices about when and how you sit and actively seeking opportunities to move differently.

Cultivating a Movement Mindset

Ultimately, this goes beyond just doing squat exercises. It is about cultivating a movement mindset – viewing movement not just as scheduled exercise sessions (though those are valuable too!), but as an essential nutrient that needs to be sprinkled throughout your entire day.

How can you nurture this mindset?

See Opportunities Everywhere: Instead of automatically reaching for the elevator, take the stairs. Park a little further away from the store entrance. Pace while talking on the phone. Fidget! Small bouts of movement add up.

Embrace Variety: While we have focused heavily on the squat, remember your body loves diverse movement.

Think about incorporating:

More Walking: Aim for consistency, and if possible, vary your terrain – walking on grass, trails, or sand challenges your body differently than flat pavement.

More Floor Living: Make your living room floor more inviting. Use cushions, low tables, or bolsters to experiment with different floor sitting positions (cross-legged, side-saddle, kneeling) while watching TV, reading, or working on a laptop. See Chapter 9 for ideas.

Reaching and Hanging: Simply reaching overhead frequently can feel great. If you have access to a sturdy pull-up bar (or even a strong tree branch!), occasional brief, passive hangs (letting your bodyweight gently decompress your spine) can work wonders for shoulder and spinal health.

Play: Engage in activities that involve spontaneous, varied movements – dancing, playing with pets, roughhousing with kids, gardening.

Listen Intently: Pay attention to your body's signals. Does your back start to ache after 30 minutes of sitting? That is a signal to stand up and move. Do your hips feel stiff in the morning? That is a cue to do some gentle mobilization stretches. Your body is constantly communicating; learn to interpret its messages.

Trusting Your Body's Wisdom

As a Doctor of Chiropractic, my passion lies in helping people reconnect with their body's inherent ability to heal and function optimally. So much of modern life encourages us to distrust our bodies – to numb pain with pills, to rely on external supports like chairs and orthotics without addressing underlying movement patterns, to accept limitations as inevitable.

I encourage you to cultivate the opposite: trust in your body's wisdom. Trust its signals. Trust its capacity to adapt and grow stronger. Trust that by providing it with the movement, nourishment, and rest it needs, you are tapping into a deep wellspring of health that resides within you. This book provides tools and understanding, but ultimately, the journey is yours, guided by your own internal compass.

Your Call to Action: Starting Today

Knowledge is power, but action creates change. As you close this book, I invite you to make a conscious choice, right now on _____ (fill in today's date) to take one small step towards a more movement-rich life. What could that be?

- Stand up right now and do five gentle supported squats
- Try the Cat-Cow stretch for one minute.
- Set a timer on your phone to remind you to take a movement break in 30 minutes.
- Decide to spend the first 10 minutes of your TV time tonight sitting on the floor instead of the couch.
- Take the stairs instead of the elevator next time you have the choice.

There Are No Cave Drawings of Chairs

Choose just one small, achievable action. Do it today. Then do it again tomorrow. Let these small actions build momentum towards lasting change.

Beyond the Chair, Back to Ourselves

Let's return, one last time, to that image of the cave wall, devoid of chairs. Perhaps its significance is not just about the absence of furniture, but about the presence of something else: a life so thoroughly interwoven with movement, with the earth, with the dynamic engagement of the human body, that the idea of needing a special object just to passively rest would have seemed unnecessary, perhaps even absurd.

By consciously choosing to move more, to sit less dynamically, and to reclaim fundamental postures like the squat, we are not trying to perfectly replicate an ancient lifestyle. We are bridging the gap between our modern world and our enduring biology. We are taking steps beyond the chair, not just physically, but metaphorically – moving beyond passive acceptance of discomfort and limitation, and stepping back towards the strength, resilience, and vitality that are our human heritage.

Thank you for taking this journey with me. I sincerely hope this book serves as a valuable guide and a source of inspiration as you reconnect with your amazing body and embrace a life of greater movement and well-being. The path is yours to walk, and your body is ready when you are.

Important Disclaimer

The information provided in these chapters are for general informational purposes only and does not constitute medical advice. Consult with a qualified healthcare professional before beginning this or any new physical activity, especially if you have pre-existing health conditions, injuries, or concerns. Listen carefully to your body; if you experience any sharp, shooting, significant, or worsening pain during or after performing, stop immediately and consult a professional. The author and publisher disclaim any liability for injuries or adverse effects resulting from the use or misuse of the information presented here.

Notes

There Are No Cave Drawings of Chairs

Bonus Chapter: The Gravity-Assisted Stretch

"There are no cave drawings of pillows or mattresses either... Our ancestors lived differently, closer to the earth."

Throughout this book, our focus has been reclaiming the squat. This bonus chapter introduces a complementary practice: a simple gravity-assisted stretch performed by hanging passively from a bar. Where squatting grounds us, this practice allows us to gently elongate, using our own body weight and the pull of gravity to create space in the spine and shoulders. It is another accessible way to tap into movement possibilities our ancestors likely experienced far more frequently – reaching, climbing, suspending – activities largely absent from many of our routines today.

Let's explore the benefits of this gentle traction, how to perform it safely, and how to structure a session for optimal results.

Dr. Chada

Why Use a Gravity-Assisted Stretch?

Allowing your body to hang passively, utilizing gravity as a gentle stretching force, offers several compelling benefits:

Spinal Decompression: This is the primary advantage. As your body hangs, gravity gently pulls your pelvis and lower body downwards, creating subtle separation between your vertebrae. This can:

Relieve Disc Pressure: Ease the compressive load on your intervertebral discs, potentially alleviating discomfort.

Promote Disc Hydration: Encourage the natural fluid exchange ("motion is lotion" principle from Chapter 4) that keeps discs healthy.

Create Nerve Space: Increase the space where nerves exit the spinal column, potentially reducing irritation or impingement.

Shoulder Health and Mobility Stretch: Hanging places your arms fully overhead, a position often neglected. This provides:

Improved Overhead Range: Helps maintain or restore the ability to comfortably reach overhead.

Gentle Stretch for Tight Muscles: Elongates muscles around the shoulder girdle and torso that commonly become tight, such as the latissimus dorsi (lats), pectorals (chest), and others, counteracting the effects of hunching or desk work.

Enhanced Shoulder Blade Movement: Allows the scapulae (shoulder blades) to glide upwards and outwards freely, promoting better overall shoulder function.

Improved Grip Strength: While relaxation is key during the hang itself, the act of holding onto the bar naturally builds grip strength over time, which is beneficial for many daily tasks.

Postural Counteraction: The overhead position and gentle traction naturally open the chest and encourage a more upright spinal posture, providing a direct counter-stretch to the slumped C-curve (Chapter 6) often adopted when sitting.

How to Perform A Passive Gravity-Assisted Stretch

The goal is relaxation and allowing gravity to do the work. This is often called a "passive hang" or "dead hang."

Find Your Support: Choose a sturdy horizontal bar. Options include a securely installed doorway pull-up bar, solid playground equipment (monkey bars), a low, robust tree limb, gymnastics rings, or a suspension trainer. Crucially, ensure it can safely support your full body weight. Test it cautiously first.

Establish Your Grip: Stand under or slightly behind the bar. Reach up and grip the bar with both hands. An overhand grip (palms facing away) or underhand grip (palms facing you) is fine – use what feels comfortable. A full grip (thumbs wrapped around) provides more security. Aim for hands positioned about shoulder-width apart or slightly wider.

Initiate the Stretch: Use a stool or bench if needed to reach the bar easily. Slowly allow your body weight to be taken by your hands, letting your feet lift from the ground or support surface.

RELAX and Lengthen (The Key!): This is where the "passive" part comes in. Let go of muscular tension:

Shoulders: Allow them to rise towards your ears naturally. Do not actively pull your shoulder blades down. Think "long arms, relaxed shoulders."

Torso/Spine: Relax your core and back muscles. Imagine your spine gently lengthening like a stretching elastic band.

Hips/Legs: Let your lower body hang heavy.

Breathe: Focus on slow, deep breaths, trying to relax more with each exhale. You should feel a stretch, primarily through your shoulders, lats (sides of your back), and perhaps a gentle lengthening in your spine. It should feel like relief, not sharp pain.

Finishing Safely: When ready to finish (based on time or grip fatigue), bend your knees and place your feet back on the ground or the stool. Release your grip carefully after your weight is supported by your feet. Avoid just dropping off the bar, especially if it is high.

Structuring Your Session: A Sample Protocol

Consistency and gradual progression are much safer and more effective than trying to hang for long periods right away. Here is a sample starting session structure:

Warm-up (1-2 minutes): Perform gentle shoulder rolls (forward and backward), arm circles, or other light movements to prepare the shoulder joints.

Gravity-Assisted Stretch Repetitions:

Duration: Aim for 10 to 20 seconds of passive stretching per rep initially. Focus on relaxation.

Rest Interval: After each rep, rest for 60 to 90 seconds. Shake out your hands, roll your shoulders. This allows your grip and shoulder tissues to recover fully before the next rep.

Number of Reps: Perform 3 to 5 reps in your first few sessions.

There Are No Cave Drawings of Chairs

Frequency: Aim to do this short session daily or at least 3-5 times per week for the best results. Consistency over intensity is key.

Progression: Listen to your body! Once you can comfortably complete your target reps and duration for a week or two, you can gradually increase one variable:

- Slightly increase the time per rep (e.g., to 20-30 seconds), keeping the number of reps the same.
- Or, keep the time the same (e.g., 10-20 seconds) but increase the number of reps (e.g., to 6-8).
- Avoid increasing both duration and number of reps significantly at the same time.

This structured approach ensures you build capacity slowly and minimizes the risk of overstraining your grip or shoulders. Remember, even accumulating just 1-2 minutes of total passive stretching time per session, done consistently, can yield significant benefits.

Modification for Comfort

If supporting your full body weight feels too intense for your grip or shoulders right away, use the Foot-Supported Modification:

Use a lower bar or stand on a stable stool/box of the right height. When you grasp the bar and relax your upper body, keep your feet (or just your toes) lightly touching the ground or stool. This allows you to control exactly how much weight you are suspending, taking some load off your hands and shoulders while still allowing you to feel the gentle upper body stretch and spinal elongation. Gradually decrease the support from your feet as you feel more comfortable and stronger.

Dr. Chada

Who Should Be Cautious? (Contraindications)

This gentle stretch is beneficial for many, but caution is advised for some individuals. Please consult with a qualified healthcare professional (your physician, chiropractor, or physical therapist) before starting if you have:

Acute or Significant Shoulder Issues: Recent rotator cuff tears, dislocations, severe impingement, labral tears, or significant, unexplained shoulder pain.

Shoulder Instability/Hypermobility: If your shoulders are prone to feeling unstable or dislocating easily.

Severe Osteoporosis: Check with your doctor regarding spinal traction, even gentle passive stretching.

Recent Surgery: Especially involving the spine, shoulders, elbows, or wrists. Clearance from your surgeon/therapist is essential.

Pregnancy: Particularly in later stages due to hormonal ligament laxity and changing body mechanics. Discuss with your provider.

Certain Medical Conditions: Including uncontrolled high blood pressure, certain heart conditions, glaucoma, or any condition where temporary increases in intra-ocular, intra-cranial pressure or increased physical activity might be a concern.

All Together Now!

The gravity-assisted stretch is a simple yet powerful tool. It offers a natural counterbalance to the compressive forces our bodies endure daily, particularly from prolonged sitting and gravity itself. It helps decompress the spine and joints, improve shoulder health, and gently realign posture.

Consider incorporating short, consistent sessions of this practice into your routine, complementing the grounding work of squatting and your efforts to move more throughout the day. By embracing both the downward connection of the squat and the upward reach of this gravity-assisted stretch, you provide more movement, helping you to reconnect with your inherent potential for health, mobility, and ease.

Important Disclaimer

The information provided in this chapter is for general informational purposes only and does not constitute medical advice. Performing gravity-assisted stretches involves potential risks. Consult with a qualified healthcare professional before beginning this or any new physical activity, especially if you have pre-existing health conditions, injuries, or concerns. Always ensure the structure you are hanging from is stable, secure, and capable of supporting your full body weight. Listen carefully to your body; if you experience any sharp, shooting, significant, or worsening pain during or after performing this stretch, stop immediately and consult a professional. The author and publisher disclaim any liability for injuries or adverse effects resulting from the use or misuse of the information presented here.

Dr. Chada

Bonus Chapter II: When You Shoes you Lose

"There are no cave drawings of pillows or mattresses either... Our ancestors lived differently, closer to the earth."

Our exploration in this book began by questioning the ubiquitous chair, prompted by its absence in the visual records of our deep human past. We have seen how returning to more ancestral postures like the squat can profoundly benefit our bodies. Now, let's apply that same lens to another modern convenience we often take for granted: our shoes.

Just as there are no cave drawings of chairs, there are certainly no depictions of structured, supportive footwear from most of human history. While early humans undoubtedly used simple coverings for protection in harsh conditions (basic wraps, hides, or sandals), the heavily cushioned, motion-controlling, often

There Are No Cave Drawings of Chairs

narrowly-shaped shoes common today are, like the chair, a very recent phenomenon in the grand sweep of our evolution.

This raises a similar question: Are these modern shoes truly optimal for the health and function of our feet, or have we, in our quest for comfort and protection, inadvertently weakened and restricted one of the most intricate and essential parts of our anatomy? This chapter explores the potential benefits of spending more time barefoot or in minimalist footwear, reconnecting our feet with the earth and allowing them to function as they were designed.

The Modern Shoe Absurdity

Consider the typical modern shoes:

Narrow Toe Box: Squeezes toes together, preventing natural splay.

Heel Elevation: Lifts the heel relative to the forefoot, altering ankle mechanics and posture up the entire body.

Thick Cushioning: Dampens sensory feedback from the ground.

Stiff Soles: Limit the natural bending and flexing of the foot.

Arch Support: Provides passive support, potentially weakening the foot's own muscular arch system over time.

While shoes offer protection, these design features can interfere with the foot's sophisticated natural mechanics, learned over millennia of navigating varied terrain without such constraints.

Why Go Barefoot (or Minimalist)? The Benefits of Grounding

Our feet are marvels of biomechanical engineering, containing dozens of bones, joints, muscles, ligaments, and a rich network of nerves. Allowing them to function without constraint can offer significant benefits:

Stronger Feet, Better Arches: Walking barefoot requires the small intrinsic muscles within your feet to work harder to support your arch, grip the terrain, and provide stability. Just like any muscle, these get stronger with use. Relying constantly on passive arch support in shoes can lead to these muscles weakening, potentially contributing to flatter arches or other foot problems over time. Barefoot time helps rebuild this natural, active support system.

Enhanced Sensory Feedback (Proprioception): The soles of your feet are packed with nerve endings constantly sending information to your brain about the texture, temperature, and slope of the ground beneath you. This rich sensory input (proprioception) is crucial for balance, coordination, and making subtle adjustments in your gait to maintain stability. Thick, cushioned shoes significantly dampen this feedback, essentially "muting" the conversation between your feet and your brain. Barefoot walking turns the volume back up, potentially leading to improved balance and reduced risk of falls.

More Natural Gait Mechanics: Cushioned heels often encourage a gait pattern where we strike the ground heavily with our heel first. While this might feel okay in padded shoes, it sends significant impact forces up the leg (knee, hip) and spine. Walking barefoot typically encourages a lighter step, often landing more towards the midfoot or forefoot, utilizing the foot's natural arch and ankle flexion as shock absorbers. This can lead to a smoother, potentially less jarring gait.

Improved Toe Splay and Function: Feet are naturally widest at the toes. When allowed to spread, the toes provide a broader base of support and contribute actively to balance and propulsion. Most conventional shoes squish the toes together, hindering their function and potentially contributing to conditions like bunions, hammertoes, or overlapping toes over time. Barefoot time allows the toes to splay naturally

Potential Upstream Benefits: As we know the body is an interconnected kinetic chain (Chapter 4), improving foot strength, sensory feedback, and gait mechanics can have positive ripple effects further up the body. Better foot function might lead to improved alignment and reduced stress on the ankles, knees, hips, and even the lower back, complementing the benefits gained from improving posture through squatting.

How to Start Walking Barefoot Safely

Transitioning to more barefoot time requires patience and common sense, especially if your feet have spent years encased in supportive shoes.

Start Slow and Short: Do not immediately go for a long barefoot hike! Begin with just 5-10 minutes at a time on safe, soft, and predictable surfaces like grass in your backyard, soft sand at the beach, or even just around your house.

Increase Gradually: Slowly increase the duration and frequency as your feet feel comfortable. Listen to your body; some initial tenderness in the muscles or skin is normal, but sharp pain is not.

Mind Your Environment: Be highly aware of where you are walking. Scan the ground for potential hazards like sharp rocks, glass, thorns, hot pavement, or anything else that could cause injury. Choose your barefoot locations wisely.

Focus on Form: Pay attention to how you walk. Aim for lighter, quieter steps. Try to land gently, perhaps more towards the midfoot, rather than heavily pounding your heel. Shorten your stride slightly if needed.

Listen to Your Feet: Build up skin tolerance (calluses) gradually. If you get blisters or sore spots, take a break and let them heal. Sharp or persistent pain means you should stop and potentially reassess or seek advice.

Keep Feet Clean: Wash your feet after walking barefoot outdoors and check them regularly for any cuts, scrapes, or embedded objects.

When Barefoot Is not Practical: The Minimalist Shoe Option

Let's be realistic: walking barefoot is not always safe, socially acceptable, or practical in our modern world. Minimalist shoes offer a valuable compromise, aiming to provide protection while interfering less with natural foot function than conventional shoes. Key features include:

Wide Toe Box: Allows toes to splay naturally.

Zero-Drop Platform: The heel is at the same height as the forefoot (no elevated heel).

Thin, Flexible Sole: Allows the foot to bend and feel the ground better.

Minimal or No Arch Support: Encourages the foot's intrinsic muscles to provide support.

Important: Transitioning even to minimalist shoes should be done gradually. Your foot muscles, tendons, and bones need time to adapt after potentially years of being supported and restricted by conventional footwear. Doing too much too soon in minimalist shoes can lead to injury (like stress fractures or tendonitis). Start with short walks and slowly increase duration and intensity.

Who Needs to Be Extra Cautious?

While beneficial for many, barefoot walking or switching to minimalist shoes requires extra caution or may not be advisable for certain individuals:

Diabetes or Peripheral Neuropathy: Reduced sensation in the feet significantly increases the risk of unnoticed injuries becoming infected. Consult closely with your physician or podiatrist before making any changes to footwear or going barefoot.

Significant Structural Foot Deformities: Certain pre-existing conditions might require specific footwear or support. Professional medical advice is crucial.

Open Wounds, Sores, or Infections: Avoid barefoot walking until any skin issues on the feet are fully healed.

Acutely Injured Foot or Ankle: Allow injuries to heal completely before stressing the foot with barefoot activity or minimalist shoes.

Unsafe Environments: Clearly, avoid going barefoot where there are obvious risks of cuts, burns, infections, or other hazards.

Almost done...

Just as questioning the chair can unlock benefits for our hips and spine, questioning our footwear can unlock the potential of our amazing feet. Allowing our feet to feel the ground, to move more naturally, and to build their own intrinsic strength – whether fully barefoot in safe environments or through thoughtfully chosen minimalist shoes – is another powerful way to counteract detrimental modern habits. It helps us reconnect with our body's inherent design and capabilities, improving function not just locally in the foot, but potentially influencing alignment and comfort all the way up the kinetic chain. It is another step "beyond the chair" – or in this case, beyond the overly restrictive shoe – towards a more grounded, resilient, and vibrantly healthy life.

The information in this chapter is for general informational purposes only and does not constitute medical advice. Walking barefoot or using minimalist footwear involves potential risks. Consult with a qualified healthcare professional (such as your physician, chiropractor, podiatrist, or physical therapist) before making significant changes to your footwear or activity levels, especially if you have pre-existing health conditions, foot problems, injuries, or concerns. Always prioritize safety: start slowly, listen carefully to your body, be mindful of your environment, and stop if you experience sharp or persistent pain. The author and publisher disclaim any liability for injuries or adverse effects resulting from the use or misuse of the information presented here.

NOTES

About the Author

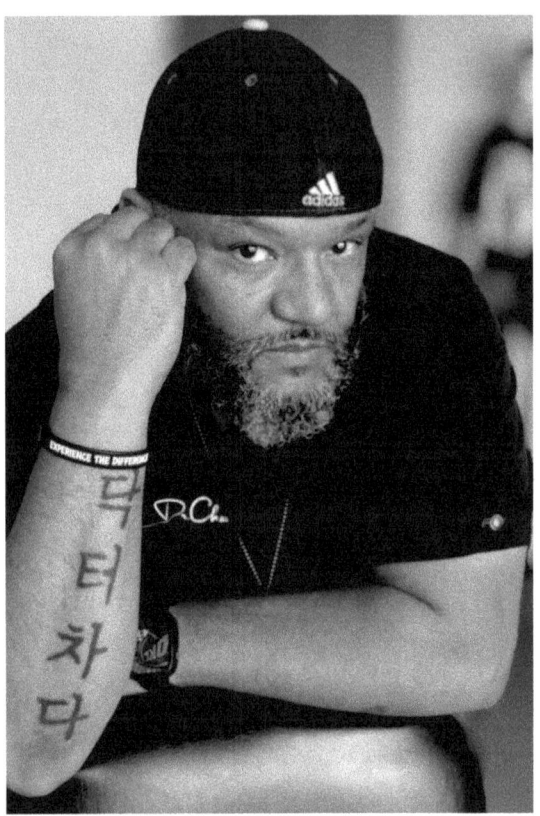

Dr. Jeremy Chada is a Doctor of Chiropractic and first-generation academic who brings a unique perspective to healthcare, having transitioned to the profession after a demanding career of over two decades as a Master Butcher. A desire for profound change after having the honor of voting for a POTUS that looked like him. Embracing "Yes We Can!" set him on a new path in 2009, culminating in his graduation from Sherman College of Chiropractic on his 42nd birthday. Prior to that was a GED, with 8th grade being the highest grade he completed before being expelled from high school.

Practicing a whole-body approach with what he has dubbed 'The C.H.A.D.A.' or The Cascading Hand Applied Dynamic Adjustment. This approach fuses his understanding of Diversified, Knee Chest Upper Cervical, Thompson, and Orthospinology techniques, combined with an abnormal passion for human anatomy as well as decades of disassembling other mammals. Dr. Chada serves his community in southern Colorado. He provides phenomenal care that goes beyond just addressing symptoms, aiming instead to uncover and address underlying functional patterns.

Ultimately, Dr. Chada considers himself just a regular guy wanting to make the world a better place. He wrote "There Are No Cave Drawings Of Chairs" to empower readers with the knowledge to question modern norms, reconnect with their innate physical capabilities, improve their health, and perhaps even find a smile along the way.

Readers interested in learning more or with specific questions related to the book's concepts are encouraged to connect with Dr. Chada. You can visit his website at www.DrChada.com or email inquiries directly to Ask@ThereAreNoCaveDrawings.com.

"In addition to treating professional athletes, rock stars and everyday people like me, I can now call myself an author."

~Dr. Chada

Appendix I - Glossary of Terms

This glossary provides simple definitions for some of the anatomical, biomechanical, and health-related terms used in this book. The aim is to help clarify concepts for readers without a background in these fields. By no means is this a complete list of terms.

A

Acetabulum: The cup-shaped socket in the side of the pelvis where the head (ball) of the thigh bone (femur) fits, forming the hip joint.

Adductors: Muscles located on the inner side of the thighs that primarily pull the legs towards the midline of the body.

Anterior Pelvic Tilt: A forward tipping of the pelvis, where the front hip bones move downward and the back (tailbone area) moves upward. Often associated with an increased low back arch and tight hip flexors.

Articular Cartilage: The smooth, white, slippery tissue covering the ends of bones within a joint. It helps bones glide easily over each other with minimal friction

B

Biomechanics: The study of the mechanics of movement in living organisms; how forces affect our bodies and how we move.

Box Squat: A squat variation where you lower yourself until your buttocks lightly touch a box, bench, or chair behind you, helping control depth and build confidence.

C

Cardiovascular Disease: A general term for conditions affecting the heart and blood vessels, such as heart attack, stroke, and high blood pressure.

Cartilage: A type of firm, flexible connective tissue found in various parts of the body, including the lining of joints (articular cartilage) and the shock-absorbing pads in the knee (menisci).

Coccyx: The small triangular bone at the very bottom of the spine; commonly known as the tailbone.

Concentric Contraction: The phase of muscle activity where the muscle shortens as it generates force (e.g., the "up" phase of a biceps curl, or standing up from a squat).

Core Muscles: The group of deep muscles in the trunk that work together to stabilize the spine and pelvis. Includes the diaphragm (top), pelvic floor (bottom), deep abdominal muscles (front/sides, like the transversus abdominis), and deep back muscles (back). Think of them as a supportive canister.

D

Deep Vein Thrombosis (DVT): A blood clot that forms in a vein deep within the body, usually in the legs. Prolonged immobility is a risk factor.

Diaphragm: The primary muscle used for breathing, located below the lungs and above the abdominal organs. It forms the "roof" of the core canister.

Dorsiflexion: The movement of bending the ankle so that the top of your foot moves closer to your shin. Adequate dorsiflexion is essential for performing a deep squat with heels down.

E

Eccentric Contraction: The phase of muscle activity where the muscle lengthens while still generating force, often controlling a movement against gravity (e.g., slowly lowering a weight, or the controlled descent into a squat).

Episiotomy: A surgical incision made in the perineum (the area between the vagina and anus) during childbirth, intended to enlarge the vaginal opening.

Erector Spinae: A group of muscles running along the length of the spine that help to keep the back straight (extended).

Extension: A movement that increases the angle between two body parts, typically straightening a joint (e.g., straightening the knee or hip). Opposite of flexion.

F

Fascia: A thin casing or web of connective tissue that surrounds and holds every organ, blood vessel, bone, nerve fiber, and muscle in place. It provides support and allows tissues to glide smoothly against each other.

Femur: The thigh bone. It is the longest and strongest bone in the human body, connecting the hip to the knee.

Flexion: A movement that decreases the angle between two body parts, typically bending a joint (e.g., bending the knee or hip). Opposite of extension.

Functional Strength: Strength that directly translates to performing everyday activities easily and efficiently (e.g., lifting, carrying, getting up from the floor).

G

Gastrocnemius: The larger, more superficial calf muscle, visible as the bulge on the back of the lower leg. It crosses both the knee and ankle joint.

Gluteal Amnesia: A term used to describe the condition where the gluteal (buttock) muscles become weak and do not activate properly, often due to prolonged sitting.

Gluteus Maximus (Glutes): The largest of the three gluteal muscles, forming the main bulk of the buttocks. It is a powerful muscle for extending the hip (moving the thigh backward).

H

Hamstrings: A group of three muscles located on the back of the thigh, running from the sit bones to below the knee. They primarily bend the knee and extend the hip.

Hemorrhoids: Swollen and inflamed veins in the rectum and anus that can cause discomfort and bleeding. Straining during bowel movements is a common cause.

Hip Flexors: A group of muscles located at the front of the hip that act to pull the knee towards the chest (flex the hip). Key muscles include the psoas and iliacus. Chronically tight hip flexors are common in people who sit a lot.

I

Impingement: A condition where structures within a joint (like bone or soft tissue) get pinched or compressed during movement, often causing pain.

Incontinence: The involuntary loss of bladder control (urinary incontinence) or bowel control (fecal incontinence).

Industrial Revolution: A period of major technological, socioeconomic, and cultural change, starting in the late 18th century, that involved the shift from agrarian societies to industrial and urban ones. Marked by the rise of factories and office work.

Intra-abdominal Pressure (IAP): Pressure generated within the abdominal cavity by the coordinated contraction of core muscles (diaphragm, abdominals, pelvic floor). Used correctly, it helps stabilize the spine during lifting or exertion.

Ischial Tuberosities: The bony prominences at the base of the pelvis that you sit on; commonly called the "sit bones."

J

Joint Congruence: The degree to which the surfaces of bones within a joint fit together. Good congruence allows for smooth movement and even load distribution.

K

Kinetic Chain: The concept that the body's joints and segments are linked together in a chain, where movement or dysfunction in one part can affect other parts up or down the chain.

Kyphosis: The natural outward curve of the spine, as seen in the mid-back (thoracic region). Excessive kyphosis leads to a "hunchback" appearance.

L

Ligaments: Strong bands of fibrous connective tissue that connect bones to other bones, providing stability to joints.

Lithotomy Position: A common position for childbirth and pelvic exams where the individual lies on their back with hips and knees flexed, thighs apart, and legs often supported in stirrups.

Lordosis: The natural inward curve of the spine, as seen in the neck (cervical region) and lower back (lumbar region). Excessive lordosis leads to a "swayback" appearance.

M

Meniscus (plural: Menisci): Two C-shaped pads of tough cartilage within each knee joint that act as shock absorbers and improve joint stability and fit.

Metabolic Syndrome: A cluster of conditions including high blood pressure, high blood sugar, unhealthy cholesterol levels, and excess abdominal fat, that significantly increase the risk of heart disease, stroke, and type 2 diabetes.

Mobility: The ability to move a limb or joint freely and easily through its full intended range of motion. Distinct from flexibility (which is just about muscle length), mobility involves joint health and neuromuscular control.

Musculoskeletal: Relating to the structures involved in movement: the muscles, skeleton (bones), joints, and associated connective tissues like ligaments and tendons.

O

Occiput Anterior (OA) Position: Generally considered the optimal position for a baby during birth, where the back of the baby's head (occiput) faces the mother's front (anterior).

P

Paleolithic: The Old Stone Age, a prehistoric period lasting from about 2.5 million years ago to 10,000 BC, characterized by the use of rudimentary stone tools and a hunter-gatherer lifestyle.

Pelvic Floor: A group of muscles forming a supportive sling or hammock across the bottom of the pelvic cavity. It supports pelvic organs (bladder, uterus/prostate, rectum) and plays roles in continence, sexual function, and core stability.

Pelvic Organ Prolapse: A condition where one or more pelvic organs drop (prolapse) from their normal position and bulge into or out of the vagina, often due to weakened support structures.

Pelvic Tilt: The orientation or angle of the pelvis relative to the rest of the body. Can be tilted forward (anterior), backward (posterior), or be in a neutral position.

Perineum: The area of skin and muscle between the anus and the vulva (in females) or scrotum (in males).

Posture: The position in which someone holds their body when standing, sitting, or lying down.

Proprioception: The body's non-visual sense of its own position, movement, balance, and spatial orientation.

Psoas: A long muscle located deep in the front of the hip and lower spine; a primary hip flexor.

Pubic Symphysis: The cartilaginous joint located at the front of the pelvis, joining the left and right pubic bones.

Puborectalis Muscle: A U-shaped muscle that loops around the rectum. It helps maintain fecal continence by creating a kink in the rectum when contracted (as in sitting) and relaxes to straighten the rectum during squatting to facilitate elimination.

Q

Quadriceps: A large group of four muscles located on the front of the thigh. Their main function is to extend (straighten) the knee.

R

Range of Motion (ROM): The full potential movement arc available at a specific joint.

S

Sacroiliac (SI) Joints: The joints located at the back of the pelvis where the sacrum connects with the iliac bones (the large, wing-like parts of the pelvis).

Sacrum: The large, triangular bone located at the base of the spine, just above the tailbone, fitting between the two hip bones.

Sedentary: A lifestyle characterized by prolonged periods of sitting or inactivity.

Sitting Disease: An informal term referring to the collection of negative health effects associated with excessive amounts of time spent sitting.

Soleus: A muscle located in the calf, underneath the larger gastrocnemius muscle. Important for pushing off the foot and ankle stability.

Synovial Fluid: A viscous fluid found within freely moving (synovial) joints. It acts as a lubricant, reduces friction, absorbs shock, and nourishes articular cartilage.

T

Talus: The ankle bone that sits above the heel bone (calcaneus) and below the lower leg bones (tibia and fibula), forming the main part of the ankle joint.

Tibia: The larger of the two bones in the lower leg, located on the inner side; commonly known as the shin bone.

Transversus Abdominis: The deepest muscle layer of the abdominal wall, wrapping around the torso like a corset. Crucial for core stability and spinal support.

Appendix II - Understanding Positions and Directions

To describe locations on the body or movements accurately, healthcare professionals and anatomists use specific directional terms. Understanding these basic terms can help you better visualize the information presented in this book. Think of them like points on a compass for navigating the human body. All descriptions assume the body is in the standard Anatomical Position unless otherwise stated.

Anatomical Position: The standard reference point. Imagine standing upright, facing forward, with your feet flat on the floor and close together, arms hanging at your sides, and palms facing forward.

Directional Terms:

Anterior: Towards the front of the body. (Example: Your breastbone is anterior to your spine). Also called Ventral.

Posterior: Towards the back of the body. (Example: Your spine is posterior to your breastbone). Also called Dorsal.

Superior: Towards the head or upper part of a structure. (Example: Your head is superior to your shoulders). Also called Cranial.

Inferior: Towards the feet or lower part of a structure. (Example: Your feet are inferior to your knees). Also called Caudal.

Medial: Closer to the midline of the body (an imaginary line dividing the body into equal left and right halves). (Example: Your nose is medial to your ears).

Lateral: Farther away from the midline of the body (towards the sides). (Example: Your ears are lateral to your nose).

Proximal: Closer to the point of attachment of a limb to the trunk, or closer to the origin of a structure. (Example: Your elbow is proximal to your wrist because it is closer to your shoulder/trunk).

Distal: Farther from the point of attachment of a limb to the trunk, or farther from the origin of a structure. (Example: Your fingers are distal to your wrist because they are further from your shoulder/trunk).

Superficial: Closer to the surface of the body. (Example: Your skin is superficial to your muscles).

Deep: Farther away from the surface of the body. (Example: Your bones are deep to your muscles).

Basic Body Positions:

Supine: Lying horizontally on your back, face up.

Prone: Lying horizontally on your stomach, face down.

Understanding these simple terms can make descriptions of anatomy, movement, and posture much clearer as you continue your journey toward better health and movement!

Pop Quiz

Instructions: Choose the single best answer for each question based on the information presented in the book.

1. What is the central premise introduced in Chapter 1 by the book's title?

    A) Cave drawings depict early forms of chairs.

    B) Modern chairs evolved directly from cave seating.

    C) Chair-sitting is a relatively recent invention, not an ancient human norm.

    D) Cave drawings show humans were primarily standing, not sitting or squatting.

2. According to Chapter 1, which very early human posture closely resembles a deep squat?

    A) The posture typically adopted during hunting.

    B) The fetal position in the womb.

    C) The way toddlers first learn to stand.

    D) Sleeping positions depicted in ancient art.

3. Chapter 2 discusses the Hadza people of Tanzania primarily to illustrate:

A) The earliest known invention of the stool.

B) A contemporary hunter-gatherer group where squatting is a common resting posture.

C) The transition from squatting to chair-sitting in modern Africa.

D) Skeletal adaptations specifically found only in East African populations.

4. What anatomical evidence mentioned in Chapter 2 suggests habitual squatting in past populations?

A) Larger thigh bone circumference.

B) Specific "squatting facets" or markings on ankle and hip bones.

C) A naturally fused lumbar spine.

D) The absence of the pubic symphysis joint.

5. According to Chapter 3, early chairs (like those in ancient Egypt or Rome) primarily signified:

A) Ergonomic design for comfort.

B) Widespread use among common laborers.

C) Status, power, and elevation above others.

D) A focus on facilitating group discussion.

6. Which invention, discussed in Chapter 3, significantly contributed to the decline of squatting as a daily physiological posture in Western societies?

A) The ergonomic office chair.

B) The automobile seat.

C) The modern sitting toilet.

D) The rocking chair.

7. Chapter 4 describes the hip as a "ball-and-socket" joint. This design primarily allows for:

A) Only forward and backward movement (like a hinge).

B) Movement in multiple directions (flexion, extension, rotation).

C) Shock absorption through cartilage compression only.

D) Stability with very limited range of motion.

8. How does squatting benefit knee cartilage, according to Chapter 4's "motion is lotion" concept?

A) By thinning the cartilage to make it more flexible.

B) By increasing direct blood flow through exercise.

C) By compressing/releasing cartilage, circulating nutrient-rich synovial fluid.

D) By permanently strengthening the menisci through static holds.

9. What specific ankle movement, often restricted in modern populations, is crucial for a deep, flat-footed squat (Chapter 4)?

A) Plantarflexion (pointing the toes down).

B) Inversion (turning the sole inwards).

C) Eversion (turning the sole outwards).

D) Dorsiflexion (bringing the foot towards the shin).

10. Chapter 5 describes the "core canister." Which group of muscles forms the *bottom* or "floor" of this canister?

A) The diaphragm.

B) The gluteus maximus.

C) The pelvic floor muscles.

D) The transversus abdominis.

11. Which muscle group, often chronically *shortened* by sitting, receives a beneficial stretch during a deep squat (Chapter 5)?

A) Hamstrings.

B) Quadriceps.

C) Glutes.

D) Hip flexors.

12. "Gluteal amnesia," as discussed in Chapters 5 and 6, refers to:

A) Forgetting lower body exercises.

B) Numbness in the buttocks after prolonged sitting.

C) Weakness and poor activation of the glute muscles due to disuse.

D) A type of hip joint impingement.

13. What is fascia, as explained in Chapter 5?

A) The scientific term for muscle fibers.

B) The fluid that lubricates joints.

C) A web-like network of connective tissue surrounding muscles and organs.

D) The nerve endings responsible for proprioception.

14. The "Sitting Disease," discussed in Chapter 6, is best understood as:

A) An infectious illness transmitted via contaminated chairs.

B) The specific type of back pain caused only by office chairs.

C) A cluster of negative health outcomes linked to excessive sedentary time.

D) Difficulty standing up due to muscle atrophy from sitting.

15. How does the typical slumped "C-slump" sitting posture negatively affect the spine (Chapter 6)?

A) It strengthens the back muscles through constant tension.

B) It reverses the natural lumbar curve, increasing pressure on spinal discs.

C) It encourages better circulation of synovial fluid.

D) It primarily strains the neck muscles but protects the lower back.

16. According to Chapter 6, how can excessive sitting impact metabolic health?

A) It significantly boosts metabolism due to constant low-level muscle tension.

B) It primarily affects digestion but not blood sugar regulation.

C) It can slow metabolism and impair blood sugar control due to muscle inactivity.

D) It improves circulation, thus enhancing metabolic function.

17. Chapter 7 highlights that squatting improves elimination primarily because:

A) It increases intra-abdominal pressure more than sitting.

B) It straightens the angle of the colon by relaxing the puborectalis muscle.

C) It strengthens the abdominal muscles needed for pushing.

D) It stimulates faster movement through the small intestine.

18. According to Chapter 7, how does squatting benefit the pelvic floor muscles?

A) By keeping them constantly relaxed and inactive.

B) By promoting optimal tone (strength and flexibility) through dynamic movement.

C) By primarily strengthening them through sustained contraction (like a Kegel).

D) By reducing their overall size and mass.

19. Chapter 8 argues that squatting or upright positions during childbirth can significantly increase the:

A) Need for pain medication.

B) Duration of the pushing stage.

C) Dimensions of the pelvic outlet.

D) Mother's blood pressure.

20. Besides squatting, what other "primal position" is highlighted in Chapter 8 as beneficial during labor, especially for back pain?

A) Lying flat on the back (Supine).

B) Sitting upright in a chair.

C) The hands-and-knees position.

D) Standing completely still.

21. What simple self-assessment from Chapter 9 helps check ankle dorsiflexion mobility?

A) The Wall Ankle Mobility Test (knee-to-wall).

B) The Supine Hip Flexion Test.

C) Measuring calf circumference.

D) Performing single-leg hops.

22. Which squat progression described in Chapter 9 involves lowering onto a chair or bench to control depth?

A) Supported Squat.

B) Box Squat.

C) Goblet Squat.

D) Deep Resting Squat.

23. What key safety advice is emphasized in Chapter 9 regarding pain during squatting practice?

A) Push through sharp pain to increase mobility faster.

B) Muscle soreness is abnormal and should be avoided entirely.

C) Sharp joint pain is a stop sign; do not push through it.

D) Focus only on breathing and ignore pain signals.

24. According to Chapter 10, the ultimate goal is not necessarily eliminating chairs but cultivating a:

A) Collection of ergonomic furniture.

B) Strict daily squatting quota.

C) "Movement mindset" and being "chair-conscious."

D) Preference for standing desks only.

25. What concept from Appendix II describes lying on your back, face up?

A) Prone.

B) Anatomical Position.

C) Supine.

D) Medial.

Email Answers@ThereAreNoCaveDrawings.com for the Answer Key

xi

Stay Connected!

Visit **ThereAreNoCaveDrawings.com** to:

Sign up for updates: Be the first to know about new articles, insights, and resources related to natural movement, posture, squatting, and holistic health.

Learn about events: Find out about upcoming workshops, webinars, talks, or local events (in Colorado, and beyond!) where I may be speaking or attending.

Access additional resources: Discover curated information, potential blog posts expanding on the topics covered in this book, and news about future projects.

Connect: Find ways to engage further with this important conversation.

Let's continue to challenge modern norms, listen to our bodies, and embrace the power of natural movement together. Thank you again for reading, and I look forward to potentially connecting with you soon!

Keep Moving,

Dr. Chada

www.ingramcontent.com/pod-product-compliance
Lightning Source LLC
Chambersburg PA
CBHW070635030426
42337CB00020B/4022